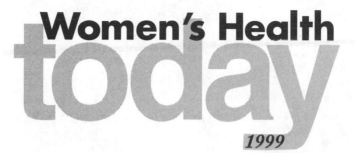

Women's Health

today

1999

Women's Health today

1999

60 Minutes to a New You

THE LATEST STRATEGIES
TO HELP YOU:

- Stay Slim and Trim
- Win at Weight Loss
- Resist Illness
- Supercharge Your Energy

**Featuring Seven Easy Quizzes
That Can Change Your Life Forever**

Edited by Susan G. Berg

PREVENTION
Health Books
for Women™

Rodale Press, Inc.
Emmaus, Pennsylvania

Copyright © 1999 by Rodale Press, Inc.
Illustrations copyright © 1999 by Narda Lebo

Prevention Health Books for Women is a trademark of Rodale Press, Inc.

Printed in the United States of America on acid-free ∞, recycled paper ♻

The credits for this book begin on page 291.

ISBN 1–57954–055–4 hardcover

2 4 6 8 10 9 7 5 3 1 hardcover

—— OUR PURPOSE ——

"We inspire and enable people to improve their lives and the world around them."

Women's Health Today 1999 Staff

EDITOR: Susan G. Berg
MANAGING EDITOR: Sharon Faelten
SENIOR EDITOR: Cheryl Winters-Tetreau
CONTRIBUTING WRITERS: Liz Applegate, Ph.D.; Mary-Ellen Banashek;
Stephen Barr; Alisa Bauman; Adam Bean; Debra Birnbaum; Chris Bohjalian;
Pam Boyer; Jennifer Cadoff; Laura Catalano; Ingfei Chen; Rick Chillot;
Erik D'Amato; Tammy Darling; Gayle Feldman; Dorothy Foltz-Gray; Marisa Fox;
Stephen C. George; Ron Geraci; Jessica Goldman; Laura Goldstein;
Susan Goodman; Megan Othersen Gorman; Rachel Grumman; Greg Gutfeld;
Toby Hanlon; Catherine Houck; Ruth Houston; Ad Hudler; Donna Jackson;
Janis Jibrin, R.D.; Kathi Keville; Sherry Kiser; Joe Kita; Allison Kornet;
Kristyn Kusek; Judith Lin; Maria Lissandrello; Barbara Loecher; Erica Lumière;
Jenny Lynch; Matt Marion; Michael Mason; Jordan Matus; Holly McCord, R.D.;
Mike McGrath; Rosie Mestel; Michele Meyer; Ellen Michaud; Nancy Monson;
Peggy Morgan; Kristine Napier, R.D.; Eileen Norris; David H. Olson, Ph.D.;
Danielle Pergament; Cathy Perlmutter; Robyn Post; Laura Quaglio; Linda Rao;
Mark Remy; Carin Rubenstein, Ph.D.; Maureen Sangiorgio; Sarah Schafer;
Susan C. Smith; Laurence Roy Stains; Michele Stanten; Alexandra Stevens;
James Sturz; Carol Tannenhauser; Margo Trott; Jennifer Tung; Densie Webb, R.D.,
Ph.D.; Yun Lee Wolfe, Mariah Yeager
ASSISTANT RESEARCH MANAGER: Anita C. Small
LEAD RESEARCHER: Sandra Salera Lloyd
BOOK RESEARCHERS: Carol J. Gilmore, Grete Haentjens
PERMISSIONS COORDINATOR: Grete Haentjens
SENIOR COPY EDITORS: Amy K. Kovalski, Karen Neely
ART DIRECTOR: Darlene Schneck
COVER DESIGNER: Lynn N. Gano
BOOK DESIGNERS: Christopher R. Neyen, Christopher Stengel
LAYOUT DESIGNER: Faith Hague
MANUFACTURING COORDINATORS: Brenda Miller, Jodi Schaffer, Patrick T. Smith
OFFICE MANAGER: Roberta Mulliner
OFFICE STAFF: Julie Kehs, Suzanne Lynch, Mary Lou Stephen

RODALE HEALTH AND FITNESS BOOKS
VICE PRESIDENT AND EDITORIAL DIRECTOR: Debora T. Yost
EXECUTIVE EDITOR: Neil Wertheimer
DESIGN AND PRODUCTION DIRECTOR: Michael Ward
MARKETING MANAGER: Melanie Dexter
RESEARCH MANAGER: Ann Gossy Yermish
COPY MANAGER: Lisa D. Andruscavage
PRODUCTION MANAGER: Robert V. Anderson Jr.
ASSOCIATE STUDIO MANAGER: Thomas P. Aczel
MANUFACTURING MANAGERS: Eileen F. Bauder, Mark Krahforst

JoAnn E. Manson, M.D., Dr.P.H.

Associate professor of medicine at Harvard Medical School and co-director of women's health at Brigham and Women's Hospital in Boston

Mary Lake Polan, M.D., Ph.D.

Professor and chairman of the department of gynecology and obstetrics at Stanford University School of Medicine

Elizabeth Lee Vliet, M.D.

Clinical associate professor in the department of family and community medicine at the University of Arizona College of Medicine and founder and medical director of HER Place: Health Enhancement and Renewal for Women, both in Tucson

Lila Amdurska Wallis, M.D., M.A.C.P.

Clinical professor of medicine at Cornell University Medical College in New York City, past president of the American Medical Women's Association (AMWA), founding president of the National Council on Women's Health, director of continuing medical education programs for physicians, and master and laureate of the American College of Physicians

Carla Wolper, R.D.

Nutritionist and clinical coordinator at the Obesity Research Center at St. Luke's/Roosevelt Hospital Center in New York City and nutritionist at the Center for Women's Health at Columbia-Presbyterian Eastside in New York City

Contents

part four

Nutrition Know-How

part five

Inner Strength

Introduction

American women are leading a revolution—a *self-care* revolution. As recently as a generation ago, women typically didn't worry too much about their health until something went wrong or until pregnancy prompted them to pay closer attention to what they ate. Now, they want to know everything they possibly can about their health. Women facing pregnancy for the first time buy every pregnancy book they can get their hands and research childbirth as if they're studying for a doctorate. The same is true with parenting. At midlife, the demand for information surges even higher. Menopause has become a cottage industry. And when it comes to topics like breast health, osteoporosis, diabetes, and other pressing issues, not a day goes by when women aren't faced with yet another breakthrough, controversy, or policy change.

No two women are alike, though. So how do you figure out how all this information applies to you?

That's where *Women's Health Today 1999* comes in. In just 60 minutes—the time it takes to finish the seven quizzes that introduce the sections—you can pinpoint the health issues that are most critical to your individual circumstances. What your mother's medical history can and cannot predict about your health status. The surprising link between moods and heart health. Why your family may be sabotaging your weight-loss efforts. Plus numerous other personal factors.

After taking the quizzes, you can fast-forward to the chapters that most closely meet your needs. Bone-saving strategies geared toward your age—20, 30, 40, 50, or beyond. Resourceful self-care strategies to help you beat allergies, headaches, stress, and insomnia without relying on bothersome drugs. How to lose weight without resorting to dangerous diet pills. And much, much more.

The quizzes are a handy way to customize health news to your needs and to prioritize on your own terms. Then you can focus on the day-to-day action strategies that make sense for *you*.

Sharon Faelten

Sharon Faelten,
Managing Editor
Prevention Health Books for Women

part one

Health Defense for Women

1

Quick Quiz

The twentieth century has produced the most amazing advances in medicine and science. We have tools and techniques for healing the body and preventing disease that even 50 years ago would have seemed nothing more than science fiction.

The downside, of course, is that health information changes so rapidly—especially as it pertains to women. As a result, you may be missing out on knowledge that is crucial to your long-term well-being.

To test your health know-how, mark each of these statements "true" or "false." Then compare your answers with those following the quiz.

_____1. While some women develop high blood pressure, it is primarily a man's problem.

_____2. All women over age 18 should have a Pap test each year, even if they're celibate.

_____3. Hysterectomy is the best solution for heavy menstrual bleeding.

_____4. A mammogram is necessary only if breast cancer runs in your family.

_____5. If you have an annual mammogram, you can skip monthly breast self-exams.

_____6. Your body stops building bone around age 30.

_____7. Hormone replacement therapy after menopause lowers your risk of heart disease and keeps your bones strong.

_____8. Despite all the new medicines on the market, aspirin remains the best choice for headaches.

Answers

1. False. About one in four women between the ages of 35 and 55 has high blood pressure. After age 55, that rate rises to one in two. Left

unchecked, high blood pressure can lead to heart disease, stroke, or kidney failure.

2. True. Celibacy doesn't protect against cervical dysplasia, the abnormal changes in cervical cells that are sometimes a precursor to cancer. A Pap test can spot these changes early, before they become problematic. (To learn more about Pap tests, see Nine Medical Tests Every Woman Needs on page 11.)

3. False. Heavy bleeding accounts for about one-fifth of all hysterectomies. Yet the bleeding can often be controlled with other, less invasive measures, including nonsteroidal anti-inflammatory drugs (NSAIDs). Most experts agree that other, noninvasive treatments should be tried before resorting to surgery. (For more information about when hysterectomy is—and isn't—appropriate, turn to When Hysterectomy Isn't Necessary on page 32.)

4. False. While heredity plays a role in breast cancer, other factors also raise your risk. Among them are a poor diet, smoking, and not having children. All women should have an annual mammogram beginning at age 40, regardless of their family histories.

5. False. Regular breast self-exams play an indispensable role in the early detection of breast cancer. The procedure itself is very easy to learn. (Be sure to read Breakthroughs in Breast Health on page 47.)

6. True. Once you reach your thirties, you begin losing about 1 percent of your bone mass every year. Fortunately, you can do a lot to preserve the bone you have. Among the most important strategies are getting enough calcium and vitamin D, and exercising regularly. (For more, check out The Latest Strategies for Stronger Bones on page 64.)

7. True. But while hormone replacement therapy (HRT) protects against heart disease and osteoporosis, it also appears to raise the risk of breast cancer. Scientists are hoping that a new estrogen-like drug, called raloxifene, will change that. (To learn more about it, read Hormone Replacement Update on page 26.)

8. False. Acetaminophen actually does a better job on headaches. Aspirin and ibuprofen, on the other hand, work best for inflammation. (To find out which medicines you should keep on hand, see Overhaul Your Medicine Cabinet on page 19.)

1

Health News from the Twenty-First Century

In this fast-paced age, one year can yield a remarkable crop of major medical advances. Imagine, then, what astounding breakthroughs lie ahead over the next 25 years. Even today, researchers are unraveling the molecular mechanisms that cause cancer, heart disease, and even aging. They've already cloned animals and made paralyzed mice walk. Here's a preview of what lies ahead.

You'll Never Have a Heart Attack

With a little exercise and temperance, your ticker can be a Timex. "Your heart could go at least 120 years," says Rodman Starke, M.D., senior vice president of science and medicine at the American Heart Association National Center. Most hearts never approach this age because atherosclerosis progresses unchecked.

Doctors hope that by 2010, they'll be able to spot faint signs of heart disease in young people. Such early detection should allow ample time to deter the disease. And people with chronic atherosclerosis may benefit from gene therapy, a process in which physicians replace the gene that makes a body more likely to accumulate artery-clogging plaque.

"Researchers can already put a corrected gene into mice and double their level of HDL (good) cholesterol," says Dr. Starke. "They may do the same in humans within 10 years."

A New Pill for Guys

Drumroll, please . . . researchers have developed a male contraceptive that works—and it should be available within three to five years, according to William J. Bremner, M.D., Ph.D., professor and chief of medicine at the University of Washington in Seattle. Indeed, in a recent major clinical trial of 300 men who were given a male contraceptive (a weekly injection of testosterone, which turns off the hormones responsible for sperm production without affecting sexual functioning), the injections were 97 percent effective. "It is five times better than the condom, better than the diaphragm, and as successful as the female Pill," says Dr. Bremner. But since it's doubtful guys will flock to the doctor's office to roll up their sleeves (especially to have their sperm counts reduced), researchers are working to develop a pill before making the contraceptive available (though getting guys to swallow that may be difficult, too).

Within 25 years, outpatient surgeries may remove arterial plaque, and cloned animals could provide a steady supply of valves and hearts that won't be rejected by the body.

But to you, it might not matter. "Bypasses, angioplasties, and heart transplants may be rare as we approach 2020," predicts Dr. Starke, "because most people will already have avoided heart disease."

What you can do right now: If you become a heart patient who needs a bypass or a heart-valve repair or replacement, be sure to ask your doctor about a new, less-invasive form of open-heart surgery, says Marianne Legato, M.D., associate professor of clinical medicine at Columbia University College of Physicians and Surgeons in New York City and author of *The Female Heart*. This procedure, sometimes called the mini-CABG (for coronary artery bypass graft), relies on the insertion of a small viewing and operating instrument. That means a 3- to 4-inch scar instead of a 12-inch one, a faster recovery time (two to three weeks instead of two months for some), and a lower hospital bill. The gentler surgery has understandably been growing in popularity for the past two years and has been performed nationwide on hundreds of people. Another advantage: Because surgeons don't have to stop the heart during the procedure, it's safer for those who are very sick.

Another interesting development in the fight against heart disease is the discovery that dental floss could save your life. A large study at the University of North Carolina further validated what much other research had already hinted at: Periodontal disease is a risk factor for heart disease. So what's the connection between your heart and your mouth? The pockets formed when sick gums pull away from teeth "have one of the highest concentrations of bacteria in the body," says Dominick DePaola, D.D.S., Ph.D., president of Baylor College of Dentistry in Dallas. Gum disease is an infectious disease, and the infection can result in bacteria being pumped into the bloodstream, which may damage the heart walls or valves. The bacteria may also cause the release of substances that encourage the formation of clots, which can lead to heart attacks and strokes.

So keep up your flossing, which helps stop gum disease. "The head is connected to the rest of the body. So when you prevent disease in one place, like the mouth, it has all kinds of important consequences for overall health and well-being," says Dr. DePaola.

You'll Be Able to Stop Worrying about Cancer

Cancer kills more than 1,500 Americans every day. But this will change in the next 25 years. "The advances in fighting cancer will be phenomenal," says Edison Liu, M.D., director of the division of clinical sciences at the National Cancer Institute. Here are six promising developments that should take the bite out of the Big "C."

1. Early detection. Within 15 years, researchers hope to be using extremely sensitive tests of blood, urine, and saliva to detect the slightest traces of cancer proteins, says David S. Ettinger, M.D., associate director for clinical affairs and professor of oncology and medicine at Johns Hopkins Oncology Center in Baltimore. Many cancers will be diagnosed, treated, and cured years earlier than they are now.
2. Vaccines. "We'll fortify the immune system with cells that can home in on certain cancers and kill them," explains Dr. Liu. "Vaccines for liver cancer, lymphomas, and melanoma may be developed within two decades."
3. Molecular drugs. By 2015, physicians will use drugs that block only the particular molecules that allow certain cancer cells to grow. "While chemotherapy acts like an atomic bomb, the newer cancer drugs will make surgical strikes," says Dr. Liu.
4. Tumor-strangling agents. "Drugs that stop cancer from forming new blood vessels are working in the lab right now," says Mario Sznol, M.D., a physician in the cancer-therapy evaluation program at the National Cancer Institute. "These antiangiogenic agents starve tumors to death." Such drugs may significantly reduce cancer deaths—and even halt advanced cancers—as early as 2010.
5. Killer genes. Gene therapy can be used to fight cancer, too, says Dr. Liu. Snuffing out the cancer-causing genes in colon and pancreatic cells—or

introducing kamikaze genes that direct the malignant cells to die—may short-circuit the disease by 2015.

6. Education. Cancer researchers seem to universally agree that getting the message out about the hazards of smoking is imperative. "Throw every other medical breakthrough out the window," says Dr. Liu. "If people stop smoking today, that'll be the most significant public health event of the twenty-first century."

Strokes Won't Be As Devastating

When a blockage, blood clot, or other circulatory problem cuts off the supply of blood to a region of the brain, it can die, thus severely reducing your ability to talk, walk, or see. Unfortunately, strokes will still threaten humans 25 years from now, but they'll be treated with much greater speed, precision, and effectiveness.

"By 2020, we'll put patients in hyperbaric oxygen cooling chambers and administer neuro-protective drugs that preserve brain tissue before irreversible damage occurs," says Sidney Starkman, M.D., an emergency physician and neurologist at the University of California, Los Angeles, Stroke Center "We'll also guide precisely targeted drugs to instantaneously unclog the blocked artery." Translation: The now life-changing ordeal may be reduced to a fainting spell followed by four or five sick days.

What you can do right now: Researchers at some of the nation's most prominent medical schools, including Harvard, Johns Hopkins, and Duke, developed and tested a diet they say could quickly reduce blood pressure–related heart disease in the United States by about 15 percent and spare one-fourth of the people who have strokes from getting them—if everyone adopted it.

The diet is pretty basic: low-fat foods (about 27 percent fat) that include 8 to 10 servings a day of fruits and vegetables. (One serving is one medium apple, one-half cup of cut-up fruit, one cup of leafy greens, or one-half cup of other vegetables, cooked or raw.) It also includes almost 3 servings of low-fat dairy foods. (One dairy serving equals one cup.) The diet itself may not be so remarkable, but the results are as good as you would get with drugs. People with normal blood pressure who followed it lowered their blood pressure a healthy average of 8½ points. That shaves an average 5½ points off the top (systolic) number and 3 points off the bottom (diastolic) number. People with hypertension lowered their systolic number an average of 11 points and their diastolic 5½ points—all without following the standard prescriptions of cutting salt intake and eliminating alcohol. Even more astounding, the diet began lowering blood pressure within two weeks. Even the researchers themselves were surprised.

Your Mind Will Stay Sharp

It seems as if new "miracle" drugs for Alzheimer's disease are appearing every week. Yet Zaven Khachaturian, Ph.D., director of the Alzheimer's Association Ronald and Nancy Reagan Research Institute in Chicago, keeps a skeptical eye on this pharmaceutical procession. He is certain, however, that we'll make substantial progress toward beating this disease in the next several decades.

"We have good knowledge of genes closely related to Alzheimer's disease, and we have drugs that can significantly delay the onset of symptoms," he says.

There will also be better treatments for people who are already afflicted. "Neurotrophins, or drugs that promote growth of brain neurons, are working in the laboratory right now," explains Dr. Khachaturian. "Soon, we may be able to regenerate brain tissue to replace the damaged neurons."

Protective drugs that guard brain tissue against Alzheimer's disease could be available in 15 years, and soon thereafter physicians may be able to correct the damage done by the Alzheimer's gene.

What you can do right now: Scientists at Columbia University in New York City and other centers gave 341 people with midstage Alzheimer's disease high doses (2,000 international units) of vitamin E. The vitamin seemed to slow deterioration by 25 percent, mainly in the ability to do everyday tasks, like dress, cook, and eat. And it delayed entrance to nursing homes by an average of seven months. Memory and comprehension didn't improve, but the evidence of benefit was strong enough to compel the American Psychiatric Association to include a recommendation for vitamin E use in its latest Alzheimer's guidelines. You don't need to take the amount of vitamin E used in the study, however. Stick with 100 to 400 international units (IU) daily. If you are considering taking amounts above 200 IU, discuss this with your doctor first. One study using low-dose vitamin E supplements showed an increased risk of hemorrhagic stroke.

Adult-Onset Diabetes Will Be Easily Controlled

Sugar can be lethal to the millions of older adults who develop adult-onset diabetes. Even when treated, fluctuating blood sugar levels can cause heart disease, blindness, dementia, kidney failure, and loss of limbs over time.

First, people with diabetes won't need to inject themselves anymore. "We'll have insulin pills and inhalers within a few years," says Richard Marchase, Ph.D., director of the diabetes interdisciplinary research program at the University of Alabama in Tuscaloosa. And "a small, biomechanical device that regulates blood sugar may be developed within two decades," he says.

Within 25 years, physicians may routinely use gene therapy to regenerate the insulin-producing pancreatic cells or force other cells to produce insulin.

Pancreatic cell transplants (much safer than substituting a new organ) with bio-engineered animal tissue are also coming, as is an artificial pancreas.

What you can do right now: The American Diabetes Association (ADA) issued three lifesaving proclamations recently: The organization revised the definition of the disease to help detect it earlier; it identified a way to spot diabetes while you may still be able to stifle it; and it stipulated when and how often to screen for the disease's mute beginning.

Adult-onset diabetes may creep up slowly, and it most often comes from putting on weight around the middle. Fortunately, the ADA's new threshold numbers will help you take preventive action more quickly. The new glucose figure that defines diabetes is 126 milligrams per deciliter (mg/dl) of blood (down from 140). Blood sugar levels from 110 to 125 mg/dl are now flagged as a condition called impaired fasting glucose. Sticking to a sensible, low-fat diet and exercising regularly may help prevent the monster from even showing its face and may keep you healthier longer.

The new ADA test guidelines recommend a fasting plasma glucose (FPG) test every three years after the age of 45. The test is inexpensive and simple. People with risk factors for the disease (especially family history of the disease, high blood pressure, lack of exercise, and being overweight) need to start screening even earlier. As it is now, doctors don't diagnose diabetes in many people until they have had it for seven or more years, and that's too much time for the disease to attack your blood vessels and organs.

You'll Never Feel Stiff in the Morning

Osteoarthritis causes joint cartilage deterioration in half of all people older than 65, sometimes making walking—or even shaking hands—excruciating. Luckily, your grip will remain viselike forever.

Within 20 years, doctors will clone the cells that produce healthy cartilage (called chondrocytes) and transplant them into joints. This procedure could render most people with arthritis pain-free. "Chondrocyte transplantation will treat certain types of osteoarthritis in patients with localized cartilage deterioration," says Daniel E. Furst, M.D., director of arthritis clinical research at Virginia Mason Medical Center and the University of Washington at Seattle.

You'll Never Have to Say "Huh?"

Almost all adults experience some loss of functional hearing with age. Someday, though, hearing aids may become as obsolete as eight-track tape players.

"Birds and reptiles regenerate their damaged cochlear-hair cells," explains

Thane Cody, M.D., of Ponte Vedera, Florida, medical director of the Deafness Research Foundation. "By 2020, we hope to have gene therapy that will regenerate cochlear-hair cells in humans, too." This will reverse most age-related hearing loss.

You'll Be Able to Smile Brilliantly

You can expect to keep 32 teeth your entire life. "In 20 years, tooth decay and gum disease will be practically nonexistent," says Irwin Mandel, D.D.S., professor emeritus at the Columbia University School of Dental and Oral Surgery in New York City. Daily brushing and flossing, fluorides, and the use of plastic dental sealants almost guarantee that you'll never spit out an incisor. But more technological armor is coming. Within 15 years, dentists will fuse tooth enamel crystals with lasers to make them impervious to decay-producing acids from bacteria. And mouthwashes spiked with antibacterial and anti-inflammatory agents will tame even extreme cases of gum disease.

You'll Still Be One of a Kind

Based on the attention given those cloned Scottish sheep, some people are convinced that scientists will routinely duplicate human beings soon. The typical plan is to ghoulishly create one body double for reserve parts and another doppelganger to send to work while you snooze.

Interesting. Spooky. But not likely.

"Cloning technology will remain way too risky to involve humans for perhaps another 50 years or so," says Arthur Caplan, Ph.D., director of the Center for Bioethics at the University of Pennsylvania in Philadelphia. And what about that sheep they cloned back in 1997? "They created hundreds of embryos, most of which died or were deformed. You want to try those odds on people?"

Scientists can reliably duplicate simple organs made of a few specialized cells, says Dr. Caplan. Heart valves? Yes. New skin for burn victims? Yes. Your next-door neighbor? No.

"It's extremely difficult to create organisms with hundreds or thousands of specialized cells from the genetic information contained in a few tissue samples," explains Dr. Caplan.

So, as always, you are unique and irreplaceable—and ready to face the next century.

Nine Medical Tests Every Woman Needs

I f you were to read what doctors read, you'd see a lot of opinions about whether testing for certain diseases is really worth it. In an effort to cut health-care costs, insurers are saying no to shelling out for many screening tests. But in many cases, it's smart to find out that you have a problem before it's too late to easily correct it.

Physicians agree. They recommend nine medical tests, each of which saves so many lives that it's definitely worth the money.

Remember that every health insurer makes its own decisions about what it will cover. And if your physician orders a test as part of her diagnosis, there's a good chance your insurer will pay. But if your insurer won't pay, these tests and your health are worth digging in your wallet for.

Note: Sometimes it pays to shop around for a lower price. Some places charge almost twice as much for certain tests as others do, as the price ranges mentioned below attest.

Mammogram

This test rates top billing, so important is it in saving lives. Many insurance plans do cover the $70 to $185 cost of mammograms, says Julie Abbott, M.D., who practices at the Mayo Clinic in Rochester, Minnesota. But maybe not

You think to yourself, "I have a yeast infection." So you do one of three things. You call your doctor, buy some over-the-counter anti-yeast cream, or wait for the itching to stop. But going to the doctor takes time and money. As for self-treatment, there's a 70 to 80 percent chance that your yeast infection is not *Candida albicans* but another kind of vaginitis— the kind that over-the-counter creams won't touch. As for out-waiting the itching, that can backfire. Symptoms may subside, but a serious infection could roar back in their place.

By the year 2000, though, you should be able to diagnose a yeast infection yourself. That's when researchers at Litmus Concepts in Santa Clara, California, expect their rapid yeast test to hit the market. Once the home test is available, you'll be able to know quickly and certainly if you have a yeast infection that's easy to treat with nonprescription medications.

The rapid yeast test is a very simple, one-step procedure that gives you almost immediate feedback. Here's how it works: A woman uses a vaginal swab to take a sample of vaginal fluid. Then she dips it into a saline solution, applies it to a test card (which resembles a plastic credit card), and waits 10 minutes. A simple, easy-to-see color change tells her whether the infection is due to yeast.

Until the test is available, though, it's a good idea to check out any vaginal infection with your doctor before you self-treat.

HEALTH FLASH

often enough. Medicare will pay for a mammogram only every other year. And for women under 65, insurance plans vary.

Who and when: The National Cancer Institute has recommended that women in their forties who are "at average risk" for breast cancer (meaning no family history) get a mammogram every one to two years. But top doctors in the country suggest mammograms every year for every woman starting at age 40.

Pap Test

Most insurers cover annual Pap tests. But if yours doesn't cover it, you'll want to pay for this essential test. Recent estimates indicate that of the women who die of cervical cancer, about half will not have had the benefit of Pap screening. So this $20 to $30 test is well worth it.

Who and when: The American Cancer Society recommends an annual Pap test and pelvic examination for all women under 18 who are or have been sexually active and for *all* women over 18. After a minimum of three consecutive "normal" test results, the Pap test may be performed less frequently at the discretion of your physician.

Bone-Density Test (DEXA)

Osteoporosis is a silent condition that strikes half of all American women over age 50. It's characterized by brittle bones that break easily, and it's known to wreak havoc on an active, independent lifestyle. The gold standard for detecting osteoporosis (through testing bone density) is the DEXA measurement of the spine and hip—a painless, quick x-ray.

While there are currently no official screening guidelines for early detection of osteoporosis, top experts in the osteoporosis field suggest that women get a baseline screening in their forties, followed by a screening about one year after the start of menopause (a time of rapid bone loss) to monitor for the debilitating condition. If your results are less than optimal, talk to a qualified doctor about tailoring a schedule of follow-up tests for you. The results from a bone-measurement test can encourage a postmenopausal woman to get estrogen replacement therapy or to begin treatment with one of the other osteoporosis therapies to prevent further bone loss, says Linda Palumbo, M.D., clinical instructor at Northwestern University Medical School in Chicago.

Medicare may or may not cover the cost of the test (although it probably will if your physician feels you are at high risk), and private health insurance plans are inconsistent in terms of coverage. The cost of the DEXA test is about $200.

Another type of DEXA test is available that measures bone density at your wrist. Called the p-DEXA, it's less expensive (between $30 and $50) and more readily available, but it doesn't measure the spine and hip, the most serious fracture sites.

Who and when: Baseline screening for osteoporosis is recommended for a woman in her forties, and it should be performed earlier if she has one or more risk factors for osteoporosis (such as a family history). That screening should be followed up about one year after the start of menopause. All women who are past menopause and have never had a bone density measurement should be tested.

Electrocardiogram (EKG)

Every adult patient who walks through the office door of Marianne Legato, M.D., for the first time can expect to get a baseline EKG, a test that measures the electrical activity of the heart muscle. "And that's the minimum in the ab-

Is It Serious?

Something hurts—your belly, your head, your knee. A painless lump suddenly appears, or you bleed a little after sex. You're worried. Is it okay to wait and see if the problem will go away, or should you call your doctor?

As a general rule, you should wait no more than two weeks, says Isadore Rosenfeld, M.D., author of *Symptoms.* If a pain or an unexplained change in appetite, sleep, urination, or bowel movements lingers for that length of time, consult a doctor. The same applies for any symptoms (such as a pain, a cough, swelling, or bleeding) that go away and then return, or that slowly worsen. Acute symptoms (trouble breathing, sudden weakness or dizziness, severe pain or bleeding) require urgent medical attention. If you can't get in touch with your doctor immediately, head for the emergency room or call an ambulance.

Below, Dr. Rosenfeld outlines symptoms you should be aware of in your twenties, thirties, forties, and fifties.

Pelvic Pain

Possible cause: Pelvic inflammatory disease (PID); ectopic (tubal) pregnancy

Specifics: PID, an infection of the reproductive organs, is usually caused by an undetected sexually transmitted disease (STD)—most often chlamydia or gonorrhea. Pain may be dull but persistent, and you may have vaginal bleeding and run a fever.

With an ectopic pregnancy, the pain is low, on the right or left side. It may occur after a missed menstrual period and progressively worsen. It may also be accompanied by vaginal bleeding, cramps, and fever.

What to do: If you suspect PID, see your doctor. Infections can be cured with antibiotics, but damage to fallopian tubes can be permanent, increasing risk of infertility and ectopic pregnancy.

For an ectopic pregnancy, get medical attention immediately. If the tube ruptures, severe bleeding, even death, can occur.

Pelvic pain can have other causes, including an ovarian cyst or growth, or endometriosis. If symptoms persist, see your doctor.

Persistent Rash on Cheeks

Possible cause: Lupus

Specifics: A butterfly-shaped rash across the nose and cheeks is a clas-

sence of symptoms," says Dr. Legato, associate professor of clinical medicine at Columbia University College of Physicians and Surgeons in New York City and author of *The Female Heart*. She's concerned that coronary artery disease still isn't widely recognized as the condition that kills more women than cancer does. Her patients receive a repeat EKG every two years. Many insurers

sic sign of this auto-immune disorder, which is more common in women than men and often strikes in young adulthood. Other symptoms may include joint pain, rashes elsewhere on the body (which may worsen after sun exposure), weight loss, and fatigue.

What to do: Talk to your doctor. A thorough medical exam, including blood tests, may be necessary. Lupus occurs in two forms: It affects the skin, and it affects internal organs as well. The disease cannot be cured, but it can often be minimized with medication and lifestyle changes.

Abdominal Pain

Possible cause: Appendicitis

Specifics: Abdominal pain is one of the toughest symptoms to pin down because it has so many possible sources—intestinal gas, ulcers, gallbladder problems, or an irritable bowel, to name a few. An infected appendix typically causes pain on the right side or near the belly button. It may be accompanied by a change in bowel movements, cramping, or low fever. It may worsen progressively.

What to do: If you suspect appendicitis, seek medical attention immediately. Rupture of the appendix can cause serious bleeding, infection, and even death. Other pains should be investigated if they persist, worsen, or continue to worry you.

Irregular Heartbeat

Possible cause: Palpitations are very common and usually not serious, if you are young and healthy. They can be caused by several conditions, however, including mitral valve prolapse (a common, usually benign heart-valve condition) or an overactive thyroid.

Specifics: It may feel like a "thump!" in the chest or a skipped, fluttery, or rapid heartbeat. It may be exacerbated by stress, caffeine (from coffee, tea, chocolate, or cola), appetite suppressants, or vitamin E supplements.

What to do: Try eliminating the triggers listed. If palpitations continue, leave you short of breath, cause chest discomfort, or frighten you, consult your doctor. She may suggest further testing (such as an electrocardiogram or an echocardiogram).

don't routinely pay for a screening EKG (the cost is from $40 to $90), but Dr. Legato believes that it is well worth paying for yourself. This test can be the first clue to an abnormality in the heart's functioning, even when there are no symptoms.

Who and when: Everyone age 30 and older should have a baseline EKG.

Serum Ferritin and Transferrin Saturation Blood Tests

A little-known but largely preventable disease, hemochromatosis or iron overload disease (IOD) occurs when a person's body absorbs too much iron. Over time, this is tough on the body, since all the extra iron begins to oxidize, or "rust," putting you at greater risk for liver problems, arthritis, diabetes, and other diseases. The serum ferritin test and transferrin saturation test, which can range from $2 to $60 each, can measure the amount of stored iron in the blood.

Who and when: Let your doctor help you decide if you should have this screening. Currently, Sharon McDonnell, M.D., of the Centers for Disease Control and Prevention (CDC) in Atlanta, is spearheading a project to evaluate the potential for screening all adults, but the call for such screenings has not been formally accepted. For now, the CDC's recommendation is that women have the tests at age 18 and again after menopause. Women with chronic fatigue, liver disease, diabetes, arthritis, or a family history of hemochromatosis are good candidates for the screening.

Lipid Profile

A complete cholesterol-level screening (lipid profile) is a measurement of your total cholesterol, high-density lipoproteins (HDL, the good cholesterol), and triglycerides (another type of blood fat). From this, the low-density lipoproteins (LDL, the bad cholesterol) can be calculated. A cholesterol test is not complete without a reading on your triglycerides.

These lipid profiles can cost from $12 to $60. Watch for advertisements for free screenings.

Who and when: Children of parents with high cholesterol (over 240 milligrams per deciliter) should be checked regularly after age 7. Most people should be screened every five years, if cholesterol is normal. If any of the serum lipids are abnormal, work with your doctor to correct the problem. Then get rechecked four months after starting lifestyle changes and/or medication to monitor the effect of the treatment.

Fasting Plasma Glucose Test

Also called a blood-sugar test, the fasting plasma glucose test measures the level of sugar, or glucose, in your blood after an eight-hour fast. Elevated levels of glucose can signal diabetes, which approximately 16 million Americans have, though the American Diabetes Association (ADA) believes only half are diagnosed. Catching diabetes early—and controlling it—can reduce many of its complications, including loss of vision, damage to the nerves and kidneys, and increased risk of heart attack. The ADA recently released new recommendations that lower the level at which a person is considered diabetic—so even if you were tested previously and were considered "normal," you might actually have diabetes. These guidelines were lowered because complications have been shown to begin earlier than previously thought. The test costs anywhere from $18 to $60.

Who and when: Every adult age 45 and older should be screened for diabetes. If the results are normal, the test should be repeated at three-year intervals. People at high risk for diabetes (those who are obese, have a family history of diabetes, are African-American, have delivered a baby weighing more than nine pounds, or have high blood pressure or cholesterol) should consider getting tested at a younger age, and more often.

Skin Cancer Screening

This often-overlooked screening should be performed once a year by your primary-care doctor, but Dr. Legato and others also suggest seeing a dermatologist every three years to get a really good head-to-toe skin cancer check. "They are more qualified to pick up any early signals of skin cancer and look over every area of the body," she says.

The screening can cost anywhere from $50 to $200, but the American Academy of Dermatology says free skin-cancer screenings are usually available. Remember, it takes 10 to 20 years for skin cancer to develop, so if you spent a lot of time in the sun during your teens, it's time to see a dermatologist.

Who and when: Every adult 18 years and up should see their primary-care physicians for an annual skin cancer screening.

Vision Screening

Some folks are lucky enough to have insurance coverage for a yearly vision screening by an optometrist or ophthalmologist. But many physicians agree that everyone should consider their eyes worth taking care of—regardless of who pays the $50 to $200 tab. Besides the obvious benefit of seeing well, there are other compelling reasons to get your vision screened. An optometrist can detect glaucoma in a patient, and an ophthalmologist (an M.D. with a specialty in taking care of eyes) can even diagnose diseases, such as high blood pressure and diabetes, just by examining the health of a person's retinas.

Who and when: Adults ages 40 to 64 should have their eyes checked every two to four years. People from their teens to age 40 should get an initial comprehensive exam, then be screened if there are changes in vision.

Don't Be Afraid to Speak Up

If you'd like to be screened for a condition, speak up. It's best to communicate your concerns to your doctor and see if she doesn't agree that the test might be worthwhile. "Unless it's a ridiculous request, most insurers reimburse for tests your physician agrees may be beneficial," says Dr. Legato. "And if the insurer refuses to pay for it, most physicians have no objection if you want a test and are willing to pay for it out of pocket."

Overhaul Your Medicine Cabinet

I s your medicine cabinet up-to-date? Probably not. There are more than 600 products on drugstore shelves that were until recently available only by prescription. Plus, new thinking about what to take for common ailments is changing so quickly that your favorite remedy may not be the most effective choice.

Of course, deciding what to buy from the array of over-the-counter (OTC) products now on the market is no easy task—unless you have some help from the experts. So here's what doctors, pharmacologists, and pharmacists recommend keeping on hand to treat life's minor miseries.

Allergies

Allergy relief once meant a dreaded weekly trip to the clinic for shots. And even as doctors' treatment options expanded, the pickings remained slim at the drugstore. Of course, nasal sprays or drops like Afrin were available—but if you used them for more than three consecutive days, they caused a rebound effect, making congestion worse than before. And OTC antihistamines could make you sleepy.

Maybe you can't teach an old dog new tricks, but sometimes you can trick an old dog. Translation? You can buy those same old sleep-inducing antihistamines and take them at night—when falling asleep is a good thing.

Painted Prescriptions

What's in a color? Perhaps more than you think, especially when it comes to medications.

Researchers at the University of Amsterdam looked at the findings of a dozen previous studies that examined how people respond to the colors of pills. The researchers concluded that color is a force powerful enough to influence the perceived effectiveness of medications.

In one case, medical students were told that they would receive either a sedative or a stimulant drug. They were then given either blue or pink placebos. Those taking the blue pills reported feeling drowsy and less alert about twice as often as those taking the pink pills.

These results don't surprise Earl Mindell, Ph.D., a registered pharmacist and nutritionist in Beverly Hills, California, and the author of *Prescription Alternatives*. "There are definite psychological ramifications of the colors of medications," he says. Blue is a calming color, and so it's associated with sedatives and tranquilizers. Pink is a cheery color, which might make it better suited for a stimulant.

In the late 1950s, when Dr. Mindell was just starting out as a pharmacist, there was an aspirin-based pain reliever available in three colors. The product is no longer on the market, but Dr. Mindell recalls that some of his customers would tell him that the only one that really worked was the pink pill. Others would swear by the white variety. Funny thing was, apart from the color, they were all exactly the same medication.

Drug companies spend a lot of time and money on developing just the right color, shape, and texture for their medications, says Dr. Mindell. Now we know why.

A French study suggests that when people with allergies take a 12-hour antihistamine, like Chlor-Trimeton Allergy 12-Hour, just before bedtime, they have less severe sneezing and congestion the next day. A nighttime dose seems to block symptoms, which are usually worst in the early morning, before they can reach their peak. There's also Nasalcrom, a spray that was released over the counter after 14 years as a prescription product. Effective against allergens of all kinds—including pollens, grass, dust mites, and pets—it doesn't cause drowsiness, create rebound congestion, or have any significant side effects. "You have to use the spray a week or two before you can expect relief," says John Weiler, M.D., professor of medicine at the University of Iowa in Iowa City. "I advise patients to start before allergy season begins."

Colds

We all have our pet theories on how to fight a cold, and most have been passed down for generations. Even doctors don't always agree. And let's not even mention the dizzying array of OTC products marketed to combat this particular malady. The most recent conventional wisdom? Medication interferes with the body's own natural healing system.

"That's a myth," says Jack M. Gwaltney Jr., M.D., head of the division of epidemiology and virology at the University of Virginia Health Sciences Center in Charlottesville and a leader in cold research for more than 30 years. "Toughing it out is needless and even foolish, because nose blowing, sneezing, and coughing may blow viruses into sinuses and middle ears and cause infection." But his newest research on squelching rhinoviruses suggests nose drops or sprays aren't the answer. "They're powerful—you get instant relief—but you're 'off and on' too much. When you're off, the rebound stuffiness can be worse than before you used the drops."

At the first sign of a cold, Dr. Gwaltney recommends taking 400 milligrams of ibuprofen (Advil and Motrin are two) or naproxen (like Aleve) at bedtime and breakfast to block the prostaglandins responsible for the inflammation that causes cold symptoms. At the same time, take an antihistamine containing either clemastine, brompheniramine, or chlorpheniramine for the drying effect (two are Dimetapp and Tavist-1). This formula should also reduce the coughing that can accompany a cold; if not, Dr. Gwaltney recommends a cough suppresant with dextromethorphan (like Robitussin Maximum Strength Cough or Benylin Adult Formula). But forget expectorants, which supposedly loosen mucus but have never been proven effective with colds in clinical trials. Quieting the cough is what's key, so you will sleep better at night and be less likely to spread your germs during the day. And as for the inevitable sore throat, Dr. Gwaltney says gargling with salt water is best, but when that's not possible, lozenges containing benzocaine should help.

Aches and Pains

Remember when Mom's answer to your every complaint was "Take an aspirin"?

That old cure-all has so much competition these days, a trip to the drugstore can give you a headache.

Backaches. Since most are caused by strain on muscles near the spine, ibuprofen or aspirin will inhibit inflammation and reduce pain. (Avoid aspirin if you're ulcer prone or on a blood thinner such as warfarin sodium.)

Fever. Try ibuprofen, recommends David O. Thueson, Ph.D., author of *Thueson's Guide to Over-the-Counter Drugs.*

Headaches. Generally, acetaminophen (Tylenol, Anacin, Panadol) works better against headaches than other pain relievers. It's also least likely to cause stomach irritation or gastrointestinal bleeding. But if you have a menstrual migraine, ibuprofen, naproxen, and ketoprofen (Orudis KT or Actron) often work better than acetaminophen or aspirin, says pharmacologist Joe Graedon, coauthor of *The People's Pharmacy.*

Interrupted sleep. Two aspirin at bedtime might help middle-of-the-night insomnia, according to a small study done at the Mayo Clinic in Rochester, Minnesota, which found that after four hours, a slight soporific effect occurs. But don't rely on aspirin as a sleep aid more than twice a week.

Minor sprains, strains, and tendinitis. Sports medicine experts recommend taking an anti-inflammatory (like Advil) to reduce pain as well as swelling. (See "First-Aid"on page 24 for more advice.)

Toothaches. Keep a supply of ketoprofen on hand: It kicks in precious minutes faster than other painkillers. But if it's staying power you need (if the dentist can't squeeze you in until tomorrow, for example), naproxen knocks out pain for 8 to 12 hours.

Stomach Upset

No mom's medicine chest was without Pepto-Bismol. And then there was that curious cure-all: soda. A "sugary treat" when you wanted it, a can of soda was suddenly medicine once you got a stomachache. Some moms insisted it be warm, or served with ice, or left out to go flat. Still others said it was all in the fizz. Now that you're old enough to drink soda when, where, and how you want, most experts agree carbonation isn't the way to go. But there's still Pepto-Bismol.

Constipation. "Psyllium is a natural product similar to bran, a food versus a chemical," says Malcolm Robinson, M.D., medical director of the Oklahoma Foundation for Digestive Research at the University of Oklahoma in Oklahoma City. "You are getting more fiber and lowering your cholesterol in the bargain." While taking it, drink eight glasses of water daily to prevent gastrointestinal tract obstructions.

Diarrhea. "We used to think that taking a medication to tighten up the bowel kept troublemaking bacteria in the body longer," says Dr. Robinson. "Now we think that using a product such as Imodium is safe for mild diarrhea. But if it's bloody diarrhea with fever, consult a doctor." Pepto-Bismol can also help guard against getting it in the first place. Try two tablets, twice a day.

Heartburn. Caused by stomach acids backwashing into the esophagus, heartburn can be most rapidly relieved by another old standby—antacids, which neutralize the troublesome acids. Chewables like Tums are best because they remain in contact with the esophagus longer, says Dr. Robinson. For longer-lasting relief—up to nine hours—the new acid controllers (Pepcid AC, Zantac 75, Axid AR, and Tagamet HB) prevent the formation of acid. But if you get heartburn more than three times a week, call a doctor.

Indigestion. Upset stomach after a rich meal? Go with Pepto-Bismol, says Dr. Robinson. (*Note*: Pepto-Bismol contains salicylate, so avoid it if you wouldn't take aspirin.)

Menstrual Cramps

They hurt. But with a little advance planning, they may hurt less. Take any ibuprofen product; timing is what's important for it to work its magic. "Take it four times a day, two days before your period begins, and these medications will harmlessly block production of prostaglandins, the hormonelike substances responsible for cramps," says Niels Lauersen, M.D., a gynecologist in New York City. "The challenge is to know your body well enough to be able to guess when your period is about to start. No anti-prostaglandin medication will work if it's not begun prior to menstruation." Continue to take it for a day or so.

Yeast Infections

If you've had one recently, you'll recognize a yeast infection the second time, and you can buy the remedies over the counter. These medications, standard gynecological treatment for decades, are very safe, with no known drug interactions and virtually no side effects (though they do dilute the effectiveness of spermicides).

The only big danger is an erroneous self-diagnosis. In one study, Temple University School of Medicine researchers found that fewer than 28 percent of women treating themselves with antifungals actually had yeast infections. The remainder had other types of infections against which anti-yeast products are useless, such as gonorrhea, trichomoniasis, nonspecific vaginitis, or vaginal discharge with no microorganisms present. So don't guess. Use an OTC, anti-yeast preparation only if you have previously been diagnosed with a yeast infection and are certain that it has returned, advises Dr. Lauersen. And if the symptoms don't subside after two or three days on an OTC medication, see a doctor.

First-Aid

For emergencies, you'll want to stock up on these must-have supplies.

Bug bites and itchy spots. One-percent hydrocortisone cream reduces inflammation and swelling by constricting affected blood vessels. It's more effective than creams that rely only on anesthetics such as benzocaine, according to *What Do I Take?*, an educational publication in which a panel of the American Pharmaceutical Association recommends Cortaid Maximum Strength.

To reduce swelling from an insect sting, apply hydrocortisone cream during the day and take an oral antihistamine such as Benadryl at night. It is important to note that massive swelling (if the entire arm versus just the bite area puffs up, for example), along with nausea, dizziness, or troubled breathing, could be an allergic reaction and needs emergency treatment.

One other note: Although OTC hydrocortisone cream is approved by the Food and Drug Administration for more serious itchy skin conditions, such as eczema and psoriasis, these are chronic conditions and should be attended to by a doctor. Never use hydrocortisone cream on chickenpox lesions or on a fungal infection such as athlete's foot.

Cuts and scrapes. Cells regenerate faster when they're moist, according to Bruce Mast, M.D., director of the Shands University of Florida Wound Clinic in Gainesville. Wash the injury gently with mild soap and water, then apply a triple antibiotic ointment or cream, such as Neosporin or Polysporin, and cover with an adhesive bandage. Do this two or three times a day until a scab forms; reapply ointment after bathing so that the wound doesn't dry out. After cuts have healed to the pink stage, Dr. Mast recommends applying a moisturizing lotion, like Lubriderm or Eucerin, to help lessen scarring.

Minor burns. Hold the burn under cool (not icy) running water for a few

Throw Away That Douche

Don't douche, say the authors of a new study that offers convincing evidence that douching may put a woman's health at risk. Researchers at the Mount Sinai School of Medicine in New York City examined the results of 30 years' worth of published research on the topic. They found that women who douched had a 73 percent greater risk of pelvic inflammatory disease and a 76 percent greater risk of having an ectopic pregnancy than women who did not.

"We don't recommend douching," says study co-author A. George Thomas, M.D. "From a scientific point of view, there's no benefit to it." Some women are reluctant to give up this practice, especially if its importance was impressed upon them by their mothers. In such cases, Dr. Thomas counsels his patients to do it infrequently (once a month or less) and never in the middle of the menstrual cycle (when there's a greater likelihood that douching will introduce harmful bacteria into the body).

minutes, which acts as a temporary painkiller. After the stinging subsides, pat dry, apply antibiotic ointment, and bandage, as with a cut or scrape.

Poison ivy. Try Tecnu to block rash formation. If you've touched poison ivy (or poison oak), wash the area with this cleanser, which was formerly sold in camping supply stores but now is also available in drugstores. It can help prevent the rash if used before it appears. If you end up with a rash, the best product is 1 percent hydrocortisone cream.

Strains, sprains, and bruises. Keep cold gel packs in the freezer for immediate use. Cooling shrinks blood vessels and helps prevent swelling, which stretches tissues and interferes with healing. Generally, sports medicine experts recommend applying ice for about two days after an injury; every two waking hours would be ideal. Apply it for no longer than 10 minutes at a time on non-fatty areas, such as knees or ankles, where nerves are near the surface and can be damaged by prolonged exposure to cold. Since fat provides insulation, ice can be applied to well-padded areas for 20 minutes. Don't place the pack directly on your skin; either keep moving it or wrap it in a thin towel, and remove it if your skin feels numb.

Hormone Replacement Update

It's enough to make your head spin.

You've heard, of course, that taking estrogen after menopause could keep your bones strong and lower your risk of heart disease. But that's not all you've heard. The same hormone, more and more scientists agree, could betray you by increasing your chances of developing breast cancer.

There you sit, trying to weigh the costs and benefits—and wishing that you didn't have to. How much easier the decision would be if there were something you could take after menopause that would protect your heart and bones without the breast cancer worry. "It would almost make the decision a no-brainer," says Nananda Col, M.D., a physician and menopause researcher at New England Medical Center in Boston.

Now one pharmaceutical company believes that it has developed the menopause "dream drug." It's called raloxifene, and it's one of a batch of chemicals known as selective estrogen receptor modulators—SERMs for short.

Like estrogen, raloxifene safeguards sturdy bones and may well protect hearts. But while estrogen nudges breast cells to divide, thus raising cancer risk, there's every sign that raloxifene doesn't do so. Nor does raloxifene spur cell division in the uterus, which is another side effect of estrogen.

"Raloxifene is a pioneering drug. I'm delighted that it's being developed," says V. Craig Jordan, D.Sc., Ph.D., professor of cancer pharmacology at North-

Every gray-haired mom who has ever been mistaken for her toddler's grandma may get the last laugh. A new study suggests that if you can have a baby in your forties, you stand a much better chance of living to the ripe old age of 100.

Researchers at Beth Israel Deaconess Medical Center in Boston compared the medical records of 78 female centenarians who were born in 1896 with those of 54 women who were born the same year but who died at age 73. The 100-year-olds were four times more likely to have had a child in their forties than the women who died younger.

The finding doesn't mean that having an infant late in life guarantees longevity or that women should put off pregnancy, says gerontologist and lead investigator Thomas T. Perls, M.D. But being able to bear a child after age 40 without the help of fertility treatments does offer a clue that not only your reproductive system but your whole body may be aging slowly.

Women who go through menopause later produce estrogen for a longer time. The hormone may prolong life by protecting against heart problems and Alzheimer's disease, notes Dr. Perls. So the study offers indirect evidence of the benefits of hormone replacement therapy. But since taking estrogen may also increase cancer risk, every woman should discuss the trade-offs with her doctor.

western University Medical School in Chicago and a pioneer in SERM research. "And the timing—right now, when there's a movement for more women's health research and more health options for women—is just right."

Better for Your Breasts and Bones

Raloxifene was approved by the Food and Drug Administration in December 1997. Excitement about the drug has been brewing ever since.

"I do a lot of talking to women's groups," says Clifford Rosen, M.D., chief of medicine and education for the Maine Center for Osteoporosis Research and Education at St. Joseph's Hospital in Bangor. "There's tremendous interest in something like this among educated women. Breast cancer—that's their big fear."

Lynnda Anido is one of the attentive ones. Ten years into menopause, she has decided to go on estrogen. "But breast cancer worries me," she says. "I have friends who've had it. It's scary, no question." Still, she has every reason to dread osteoporosis, too. Her mother fell and broke her hip while in her mid-seventies. "I live a very active life," Anido says. "I used to be a dancer, and I still teach it. I'm very concerned about bone fractures."

Bone loss after menopause is normal. The numbers vary, but a menopausal woman's bone mass can decrease by as much as 20 percent during the first five years after her periods cease. After that big decline, she continues to lose bone throughout the rest of her life, although at a much slower pace. It's no wonder that half of all women stand to fracture some bone or another in their life-times—that is, if they're not taking estrogen. If they are, the rate of fractures is halved. Could raloxifene do the same thing?

The drug's manufacturer, Eli Lilly and Company, is confident. About the time that it applied for FDA approval of raloxifene, the company released two years' worth of data from clinical trials involving 1,200 postmenopausal women ages 45 to 65. Three-fourths of the women had taken various doses of ralox-ifene, while the rest had taken placebos (fake pills). When scientists evaluated the women's bone density by measuring the mineral calcium phosphate, they found that the raloxifene-takers had increased their bone density by an aver-age of 2 to 3 percent. The placebo-takers, meanwhile, had lost bone density.

The bone gains associated with raloxifene, at least in the spine, were only about half of those associated with estrogen. But more important, the new drug kept women from losing bone, says raloxifene researcher Ethel Siris, M.D., di-rector of the osteoporosis program at Columbia-Presbyterian Medical Center in New York City. The women in the trial, she points out, didn't have osteo-porosis. So they didn't need to gain bone—they just needed to preserve what they had. "Raloxifene does the job," she says. "It's neat. It's great stuff."

Armor for Your Heart

Raloxifene may be beneficial to more than just bones. Though the findings to date aren't as definitive, research suggests that the drug might fight heart dis-ease, the number one killer of women.

Throughout the clinical trials and in a more focused study of 390 women, raloxifene lowered total blood cholesterol as well as low-density lipoprotein (LDL, the bad cholesterol), just as conventional estrogen replacement therapy does. The drug also raised high-density lipoprotein (HDL, the good choles-terol), though not as robustly as estrogen can.

On the other hand, raloxifene outdid estrogen in a comparison of their effects on two other heart disease baddies, triglycerides and fibrinogen (both of which promote blood clots). Triglyceride levels typically climb in women taking estro-gen, but they didn't seem to do so in women taking raloxifene. And fibrinogen levels, which are lowered by estrogen, were lowered even more by raloxifene.

Keep in mind, too, that raloxifene bestows its benefits without doing the dangerous thing estrogen does: promoting cell division in the breasts and uterus. "It does look promising, especially for a woman who's at increased risk for breast cancer," says JoAnn Manson, M.D., co-director of women's health at Brigham and Women's Hospital in Boston. There's even hope that raloxifene might actively discourage the growth of preexisting breast and uterine tumors, as it appears to do in laboratory rats.

Old News Is Good News

For all of their hot-off-the-press newsworthiness, raloxifene and other SERMs are hardly new. When the first of these estrogen-like chemicals was cooked up in the 1960s, researchers quickly realized that they had tapped a rich supply of potential drugs for women. "Scientists found that you could mate rats and give them one of these drugs the following day, and none of the rats would get pregnant," recalls Dr. Jordan. "It was the time of sexual revolution, so it was divined that this would be a great morning-after pill." But the physiology of rats is rather different from that of women, who responded to the drugs by releasing eggs and promptly getting pregnant. Galling, no doubt, for the women. But it did lead to the development of the fertility drug Clomid, which has helped many a woman bear the baby she longed for.

As the scientists toiled on, they speculated that SERMs could have other uses. At some sites in the body, the drugs interfere with estrogen; at others, they mimic estrogen. The tip-off came from the most famous of all SERMs: the breast cancer drug tamoxifen. Developed by Dr. Jordan, tamoxifen blocks rogue breast cells from dividing by fitting like a key into a lock inside these cells. The lock is a molecule called an estrogen receptor. While the tamoxifen key fits that lock, it doesn't turn it. Since breast cancer cells depend on estrogen for growth, tamoxifen—by jamming the lock—stops the hormone from betraying the body.

Now here's what makes the SERMs so remarkable: While they jam the estrogen lock in some tissues, they turn it or don't fit it in other tissues. This is what led scientists to begin searching for a SERM that acts like estrogen in the bones and heart but like an anti-estrogen in the breasts and uterus.

Tamoxifen, excellent as it is as a breast cancer drug, doesn't fit the bill. While it inhibits breast cell division, strengthens bones, and lowers cholesterol, it also behaves like estrogen in the uterus, slightly raising the risk of uterine cancer in those who take it. It's an acceptable risk for some women but not for others.

So in the mid-1980s, Dr. Jordan began experimenting with raloxifene. In studies with "menopausal" laboratory rats (their ovaries had been removed), the drug appeared to keep the animals' bones strong and to substantially reduce their rate of mammary tumors (the rodent equivalent of breast cancer). And when Dr. Jordan examined each rat's uterus for signs of cell overgrowth, he found none.

Some Unanswered Questions

Thus far, raloxifene seems to be standing up to the shining promise it showed in Dr. Jordan's research. Still, it is an unknown quantity—even more so than estrogen.

For example, no one knows for sure whether raloxifene really prevents fractures, as opposed to simply upping bone density (though it's likely to since it acts like estrogen). And while the drug does some good for women's heart disease risk profiles, no one knows whether that will actually translate into fewer heart attacks. "It's going to be at least a decade before we know the balance of risks and benefits for raloxifene," says Dr. Manson.

Then there are those other things that estrogen does or may do: warding off Alzheimer's disease; fighting arthritis and colon cancer; helping with a fading libido, vaginal dryness, and aging skin. All are reasons that many women opt for estrogen replacement therapy. Can raloxifene fill the bill?

Answers will come. Right now, Eli Lilly is backing a large raloxifene trial involving 7,700 women ages 60 to 75 in more than 20 countries. Initially running for three years, it will look at a cornucopia of health factors: spine fracture and breast cancer rates, mental acuity, heart attacks, strokes, and side effects.

Some side effects have already been documented. A few women taking raloxifene developed blood clots in their legs, just as a small number of women on estrogen do. Hot flashes, normally experienced during menopause, were also reported by some women taking raloxifene—and at a higher rate than in women taking placebos. Though the flashes were mild and transient, the finding does give pause to physicians like Dr. Col. She has seen a lot of patients who are dealing with menopause, and she knows what weighs on their minds. "If the drug is not making them feel good right now—even if they know it will prevent disease in the future—it's going to be a hard sell," she notes.

But it's also true that, like Lynnda Anido, many women feel stuck between a rock and a hard place. While Anido has imagined herself like her mother, housebound since that hip fracture, she hasn't forgotten the fear and the disfiguring breast surgery endured by her friends. "I will consider taking raloxifene," she says. "It eliminates the dilemma."

Making the Decision

As with estrogen replacement therapy, raloxifene isn't for everyone. Nor will it make estrogen obsolete. "But for women who fit a certain profile, it's going to be great," says Dr. Siris. Here's her advice.

If you haven't reached menopause: Raloxifene isn't for you, because your body is still making enough estrogen on its own. "Premenopausal women should just be taking good care of themselves," says Dr. Siris. "They should be doing the sensible things in life, like exercising, eating foods with plenty of calcium and vitamin D, not smoking, and not drinking to excess." But you should also be thinking ahead. "Chat with your gynecologist," suggests Dr. Siris. "Start reading and learning."

If you're bothered by early menopause symptoms: Raloxifene won't help. As mentioned earlier, research has shown that the drug can actually increase the occurrence of hot flashes. Its effects on other symptoms, such as insomnia and moodiness, haven't been studied. You may want to consider estrogen instead. Taken for up to five years, standard hormone replacement therapy doesn't seem to raise breast cancer risk.

If you're past menopause: Think seriously about raloxifene. Its power, according to Dr. Siris, lies not in short-term relief but in long-term prevention. "Suppose you're a few years postmenopausal, and you're feeling pretty good," she says. "But somebody measures your bone density because your mother broke her hip, and you find that you have somewhat low bone mass. Not osteoporosis yet, but you can see the writing on the wall if you don't take measures. And maybe your cholesterol doesn't look great, and maybe your dad died of a heart attack. These aren't unusual scenarios." Suppose, furthermore, that you don't want to take estrogen because it makes your breasts tender, or it brings on monthly bleeding, or you're scared about breast or uterine cancer.

"Raloxifene will give you a bone benefit that's quite substantial," says Dr. Siris. "It's going to lower bad cholesterol and raise good cholesterol, though not as much as estrogen would. It's going to do nothing to the uterus—you won't bleed or have malignant changes. And it does not create breast problems." It's not risk-free, however. As mentioned earlier, in rare cases, raloxifene—like estrogen—has led to blood clots in the legs. And it probably isn't the best choice if your main worry is protecting your heart, since evidence of its benefit there is still preliminary.

If you're already taking estrogen: Stay on it if you're happy with it, advises Dr. Siris. Researchers have much confidence in estrogen's bone and heart benefits. But if you've been on estrogen for more than 10 years—when cancer risk may start to rise—consider asking your doctor about switching to raloxifene. If, on the other hand, you've recently started estrogen, keep an eye on the raloxifene trials now under way, and maybe make the switch later.

If you have osteoporosis: Opt for a more potent drug such as alendronate (Fosamax), recommends Dr. Siris. Raloxifene has not yet been shown to treat osteoporosis by, for instance, reducing fracture rates.

5

When Hysterectomy Isn't Necessary

Contrary to what some doctors might tell you, hysterectomy isn't the only answer to fibroids and other gynecological problems.

The numbers are staggering. Each year, more than half a million women undergo hysterectomies, the second most common surgery in America among women of reproductive age. And it's major surgery. Recovery can take weeks or months, and as with any surgery, there's a real risk of death—an estimated 1 in 1,000 women die from this procedure.

In short, it's no small thing, and it's usually unnecessary. "About 90 percent of women who have a hysterectomy could have been offered an alternative," says Brian Walsh, M.D., director of the Menopause Clinic at Brigham and Women's Hospital in Boston. But most women are never given the choice.

Why? Some doctors don't know about the options. Today, there are safer alternatives. Virtually all involve fewer risks and a shorter (or no) recovery time. And some doctors don't mention procedures that they don't have the skills to perform themselves.

So what do you do when your doctor tells you that you need a hysterectomy? Here are three of the most common causes of hysterectomy and the ways to treat them that don't involve removing your uterus.

When Menopause Won't Wait

One in every 100 women experiences what doctors call premature ovarian failure. Many are under age 35; some are only in their teens. These women have the ovaries of a 50-year-old. They have no eggs left, or so few that ovulation is sporadic.

Like their older counterparts who go through menopause at the expected age, these young women grapple with myriad potential health problems, including osteoporosis, stroke, and loss of sex drive. In an even crueler twist, they're suddenly denied the opportunity to have biological children of their own. "Of all the diagnoses I deliver to patients," says Gerard Conway, M.D., an endocrinologist at Middlesex Hospital in London, "this is the most devastating."

But there is some good news. Dr. Conway, who specializes in the treatment of premature ovarian failure, has identified a blood test that enables a woman to determine whether she is at risk for early menopause caused by a genetic defect. For years, certain abnormalities in the X chromosome have been linked to early ovarian failure. If a girl never begins menstruating, she is given a blood test to determine whether genetics is to blame. Dr. Conway's breakthrough is to offer this test to young women with family histories of early menopause.

The test helps at-risk women by putting their minds at ease or—if the blood test confirms that they do face early menopause—by allowing them time to plan a family. A woman who knows she's likely to undergo early menopause can decide to have children sooner or consider other options, such as adoption, freezing embryos for possible future use, or finding an egg donor.

Dr. Conway hopes that more widespread use of this blood test will help physicians catch ovarian failure earlier. Until testing becomes widely available, the best way to find out whether you're at risk for early menopause is to investigate your own family history. Ask your mother and your grandmothers. If they went through menopause prematurely, you may, too.

HEALTH FLASH

Fibroids

What are they? Fibroids, or uterine leiomyomas, are bundles of muscle and connective tissue that can grow inside or outside the uterus. Not much is known about why they start, says Adriane Fugh-Berman, M.D., chairman of the National Women's Health Network, an independent consumer advocacy organization in Washington, D.C. "We do know that estrogen makes them grow, and that when a woman goes through menopause, fibroids usually shrink, unless she takes hormone replacement therapy (HRT)." Fibroids are virtually always benign. But they're the number one cause of hysterectomy (making up a third of all hysterectomy surgeries in the United States).

How common are they? About a quarter of all women in their thirties and forties may have fibroids.

What are the symptoms? As fibroids grow, they are more likely to trigger symptoms that, though not life-threatening, can sometimes make life miserable. "They can cause bleeding—in some cases, heavy bleeding throughout the menstrual cycle—leading to anemia," notes Dr. Walsh. Other symptoms include pain, frequent urination, infertility, and recurrent miscarriages.

How are they best diagnosed? Along with a complete history and thorough pelvic examination, the doctor should perform two kinds of ultrasound: an abdominal ultrasound, done from the top of the belly, to rule out the possibility of ovarian cancer; and transvaginal ultrasound, done by inserting a probe inside the vagina, to pinpoint the exact size and location of the fibroids. These are simple office procedures that don't require an incision or anesthesia.

When is a hysterectomy inappropriate? The worst reason to remove a fibroid: Because it's there. If it isn't causing any symptoms, the experts seem to agree, it probably doesn't need removal. Not even if it's big. "Doctors used to say that a woman's uterus ought to be removed when a fibroid got larger than the size of a 12-week pregnancy," says Steven R. Goldstein, M.D., professor of obstetrics and gynecology at New York University School of Medicine in New York City and director of gynecologic ultrasound at the university's medical center. "At that size, the doctor could no longer palpate (feel) the ovaries to check for enlargement that might signal uterine cancer. But nowadays, with ultrasound, we can usually see whether ovaries are the normal size regardless of the fibroid's size."

What are the treatment alternatives? Once you have been diagnosed with fibroids, there are several alternative treatments you can try.

Watching and waiting. "Sometimes I've counseled women who might be fairly close to menopause to just wait," says Dr. Fugh-Berman.

But it is a good idea to have fibroids checked regularly by a physician to make sure they're not growing rapidly. They should be checked every six months when they first appear.

After six months, says Dr. Walsh, "if a fibroid has grown from two to only

Help for Fibroids

If you have fibroids that require treatment through surgery, you want to find a doctor who's qualified to do the job. "Just because she has done tons of hysterectomies doesn't qualify her to do a myomectomy," says Adriane Fugh-Berman, M.D., chairman of the National Women's Health Network, an independent consumer advocacy organization in Washington, D.C. "It's a difficult procedure and takes a longer time to learn." Here are some key questions to ask the doctor you're considering.

1. Do you ever give a transfusion during a myomectomy? "The correct answer is no. If the answer is that most women need a blood transfusion, then you're in the wrong office," says Nora Coffey, director of HERS (Hysterectomy Educational Resources and Services), an organization that counsels women about hysterectomy.

   "I haven't given one in the last 250 procedures that I've done," adds Michael E. Toaff, M.D., senior attending physician at Bryn Mawr Hospital in Bryn Mawr, Pennsylvania. "If you have great expertise, it's very, very rare that you have to give blood."

2. Are you board certified in gynecology? Correct answer: Yes.

3. How many myomectomies have you performed? The correct answer, says Dr. Toaff, should be in the hundreds. How many have you done in the last year? "At least 50 cases a year," he says, "so they have ongoing experience."

4. How many surgeries that had started as myomectomies ended up as hysterectomies? "If it's more than 2 percent, it's too many," states Coffey.

5. Have you done many surgeries for fibroids as large as mine? Best answer: Yes, plenty.

For more information on fibroids and alternative surgery, check out Dr. Toaff's Web page, "Alternatives to Hysterectomy," at www.netreach.net/~hysterectomyedu.

---

three inches, that's not fast, and you can stretch out checkups to annually. If it has grown from two inches to eight inches, that's cause for concern." Another danger sign is new fibroids appearing or rapid fibroid growth occurring in women who are past menopause (even women on HRT).

Myomectomy. This is surgery that removes the fibroids, leaving the uterus intact. Myomectomies are becoming more routine outside of Europe—an estimated 123,000 U.S. women choose them every year—but it still can take an effort to find a physician who is skilled at the procedure.

If the fibroid is growing into the uterine cavity (submucous), the doctor can schedule outpatient surgery called resectoscopic myomectomy, notes Dr. Goldstein. "If the doctor has the equipment and the know-how, this isn't much more involved than a D and C (dilatation and curettage)." In addition, there is no incision, and there's little recovery time.

The myomectomy becomes more complicated if the fibroid is on the outside wall of the uterus (subserous) or within the muscular wall (intramural). Even so, the myomectomy can be done by using a laparoscope on an outpatient basis under general anesthesia, and pain and recovery time are minimal.

The more complex myomectomies are done with a larger abdominal incision under general anesthesia. The uterus is opened, the fibroids are removed, and the uterus then reconstructed. These are most often done on women who have many fibroids, large fibroids, or fibroids in difficult locations, or on women who plan to have children. "It entails a recovery comparable to any other major abdominal surgery," notes Howard A. Zacur, M.D., Ph.D., professor of reproductive endocrinology at Johns Hopkins Medical Institutions in Baltimore. Still, abdominal myomectomy may be easier for women than abdominal hysterectomy.

There's one big drawback to all myomectomies: Fibroids grow back in about 15 to 30 percent of women who've had one. These women may need repeat procedures—or even, eventually, hysterectomies.

Alternative medicine. Reports indicate that while alternative medicine is not very helpful for shrinking fibroids, it has helped some women control some of the symptoms.

Abnormal Bleeding

What is it? Heavy or abnormal bleeding, also called dysfunctional uterine bleeding, leads to a fifth of all hysterectomies in the United States.

What are the symptoms? To some women, it means very heavy periods; others have unpredictable bleeding throughout their cycles. In severe cases, it can lead to anemia. It is sometimes a sign of precancerous or cancerous conditions.

How is it best diagnosed? Abnormal bleeding calls for a thorough investigation, and that should start with a detailed history. The most important question: Is the bleeding cyclical, or is it unpredictable?

For women with irregular bleeding throughout their cycles, a Pap test and endometrial sampling—to look for precancerous or cancerous cells in the cervix or uterus—is vital. This means scraping some cells from the cervix, the uterus, or both. "I do it in the office, and it takes about 10 seconds and causes a little cramping," says Dr. Walsh. It's also important to do an ultrasound to locate possible growths, such as fibroids, that might be causing the bleeding. For women with regular but heavy periods, biopsy is not as vital, but an ultrasound can supply important diagnostic information.

When is a hysterectomy inappropriate? Hysterectomies are not appropriate when the cause of the bleeding hasn't been diagnosed or when medications such as hormones haven't yet been tried. Most experts agree that hysterectomy should only be considered as a last resort. According to some experts, fewer than 10 percent of cases of genuine abnormal bleeding should require a hysterectomy.

What are the treatment alternatives? Depending on the cause of the bleeding, treatments might include the following options.

Nonsteroidal anti-inflammatory drugs (NSAIDs). These can sometimes help slow down bleeding.

Combination oral contraceptives (OCs). These are often ideal for women who are not ovulating regularly and are therefore bleeding throughout the month. "OCs can give wonderful regularity," says Dr. Walsh. And they can help ward off the risk of endometrial cancer, a disease which is more likely to strike women with irregular ovulation.

Progesterone. This can be helpful for women with irregular ovulation leading to unusual bleeding. Dr. Walsh often uses it for women who don't want to take or can't tolerate birth control pills.

How does it work? Progesterone regulates the monthly growth and shedding of the uterine lining. "If you don't have progesterone," Dr. Walsh explains, "this lining gets thicker until it gets very unstable, and a little piece may fall off, and sometimes you have spotting. Other times a whole chunk falls off, and you have very heavy bleeding." Taking a progestin for 10 to 14 days can regularize the cycle. (For women who cannot tolerate synthetic progestins, natural progesterone can be a more comfortable choice. See "Taking a Different Approach" on page 40.)

Endometrial ablation. This is another alternative to hysterectomy. In this procedure, the endometrium (the inner lining of the uterus) and the basilis (the layer under it) are destroyed. "We can do it vaginally. It's a minor procedure, and you can keep your uterus," says Dr. Fugh-Berman. "It's permanent, but it's much less invasive than hysterectomy."

The success rates of endometrial ablation are good. Studies show fewer complications and much shorter hospital stays and recovery periods compared to hysterectomy.

Perhaps the number one drawback is that ablation is not as complete a solution for bleeding as hysterectomy. "No matter which ablation technique is used, a third of patients will have no more bleeding," says Dr. Walsh. "A third will have spotting or a light flow that needs a panty liner. Twenty-five percent will have average periods. And 5 to 10 percent are no better afterward than they were before." Another downside is that ablation leaves the woman infertile.

After menopause, women who've had an ablation and wish to take estrogen will need a progestin, too. That's because ablation might disguise one of the key symptoms of endometrial cancer—bleeding.

Because of the downsides, says Dr. Goldstein, many of his patients use medication to keep bleeding to a minimum and opt for neither ablation nor hysterectomy. Once they're through menopause, then bleeding won't be an issue anymore, provided they're not taking HRT.

Endometriosis

What is it? In endometriosis, bits of the lining of the uterus grow outside the uterus in the abdomen and on the ovaries. Fueled by estrogen, the tissue then grows and bleeds on a monthly cycle. This can lead to chronic pain, inflammation, scar tissue, and other problems. After menopause, endometriosis tends to go away, unless a woman takes HRT.

The causes of endometriosis are unknown, but theories include a genetic tendency; stray endometrial cells that might flow back through the fallopian tubes and settle in the pelvis; exposure to toxins; and even the possibility that it is an autoimmune disorder. Endometriosis causes about a fifth of all hysterectomies in the United States.

How common is it? As many as 20 percent of all women have endometriosis, but most have no symptoms. Once symptoms do appear, however, early treatment is very important.

What are the symptoms? Endometriosis is linked to chronic pelvic pain, especially during menstruation, intercourse, and urination; it's also linked to infertility and other problems.

How is it best diagnosed? The diagnosis is made with a laparoscopy, an outpatient procedure done under general anesthesia. The doctor inserts a slender optical instrument through a small incision in the lower abdomen to look around for growths of endometrial tissue. "We're still looking for effective noninvasive ways to diagnose endometriosis, but they're not here yet," says Tess Thompson, support program coordinator for the Endometriosis Association, an international self-help organization based in Milwaukee.

When is a hysterectomy inappropriate? A hysterectomy alone may not be considered an effective treatment for endometriosis—frequently, the ovaries have to be removed as well to help stop the endometrial tissue implants from growing. And even then, it doesn't always work. "For some women with severe, advanced endometriosis with well-documented scar tissue, sometimes a hysterectomy and oophorectomy (removal of the ovaries) have to be done, but that's in a very small number of people," says Dr. Goldstein.

What are the treatment alternatives? Endometriosis can't be cured, but it can be controlled. Here's how.

NSAIDs. These can be used for pain. A woman who doesn't respond to one type might respond to another.

Oral contraceptives. OCs alter the balance of estrogen and progesterone, slowing the progression of endometriosis, says Dr. Walsh. OCs are most effective for milder cases, he adds.

Help for Endometriosis

If you've been diagnosed with endometriosis, your first step is to contact the Endometriosis Association. This international self-help organization offers many valuable resources. To receive introductory information, you can write to the organization at 8585 North 76th Place, Milwaukee, WI 53223.

One must-have book is *The Endometriosis Sourcebook*, by Mary Lou Ballweg and the Endometriosis Association. This 400-plus page book offers the latest information on endometriosis and is available in bookstores as well as from the Endometriosis Association. The book describes conventional and alternative treatments and includes an extensive discussion of the pros and cons of hysterectomy.

Gn-RH agonists. These are powerful hormones that block estrogen and shrink endometrial tissue. The most commonly used ones for endometriosis are Synarel and Lupron. One drawback, however, is that they have powerful side effects, especially Lupron. "It's like menopause with a vengeance," says Dr. Walsh. These drugs are usually not a long-term solution—women don't use them for more than a few months, mainly because they could lose bone from estrogen deprivation.

Outpatient laparoscopic surgery. This surgery can be performed during the same procedure in which endometriosis is diagnosed. The stray endometrial growths can be destroyed with an electrical device or a laser. The disease does have a tendency to recur, but birth control pills can help maintain the regression.

Laparotomy. This procedure may be required for more extensive disease. It entails more and larger abdominal incisions, a few days in the hospital, and a longer recovery time.

Alternative medicine. Some women have gotten good results, especially when combining conventional medicine with approaches like Traditional Chinese Medicine, herbs, nutrition, supplements, and others (see "Taking a Different Approach" on page 40).

Where to Get Good Help

Your doctor says that you need a hysterectomy. You're not so sure. What do you say? "You should ask, 'Is there any procedure, short of hysterectomy, either medical or surgical, that could resolve my problem?'" suggests Michael E. Toaff, M.D., senior attending physician at Bryn Mawr Hospital in Bryn Mawr, Pennsylvania.

If you don't get a satisfactory answer, where do you turn next? Your top pri-

When You Do Need a Hysterectomy

There is one indication for hysterectomy about which experts do agree: bona fide invasive cancer of the uterus. "There really isn't a safe alternative to hysterectomy in this case," says Brian Walsh, M.D., director of the Menopause Clinic at Brigham and Women's Hospital in Boston. For most cases of invasive cancer of the cervix and ovaries, a hysterectomy is usually needed, too. That's because those cancers usually spread through the uterus. The exception is if you have very early cervical cancer and are determined to keep your uterus. The option then is extensive cone biopsy, which involves removal of the affected areas. Talk to your physician about it.

Invasive cancer is different from precancers of the cervix and uterus, points out Dr. Walsh. Precancers of the cervix can be treated with local surgery, and uterine precancers can be treated with hormones. "Often, hormones work, but if not, a hysterectomy might be needed later," he says.

ority, all the experts agree, should be to find a physician or surgeon who is experienced and skilled in the alternatives you are considering. How?

❖ Try a teaching hospital for a second opinion or treatment. A Canadian study showed that health care providers who are affiliated with teaching hospitals perform hysterectomy less often than providers who are not affiliated with teaching hospitals. "They have access to the latest medical technology and research," says Dr. Zacur.

❖ Contact HERS (Hysterectomy Educational Resources and Services). This pioneering organization is an invaluable resource for a woman determined to keep her uterus. "We counsel each woman individually depending on her history and tell her her options," says Nora Coffey, director. They can also provide names of skilled physicians in your region. You can write to HERS at 422 Bryn Mawr Avenue, Bala Cynwyd, PA 19004.

Taking a Different Approach

Practitioners of herbal and alternative therapies believe that their healing techniques can benefit many conditions traditionally treated with hysterectomy. Here are the most—and least—effective natural approaches, according to Dr. Fugh-Berman and Tori Hudson, N.D., a naturopathic physician and professor at the National College of Naturopathic Medicine in Portland, Oregon.

Bleeding. "Natural therapies are almost always successful for bleeding," says Dr. Hudson. A careful diagnosis by a medical practitioner is always important, she adds. Once a diagnosis is established, Dr. Hudson may use the following therapies.

Natural progesterone. "This is the most reliable method," says Dr. Hudson. It can regularize the menstrual cycle and prevent endometrial overgrowth—and it may have fewer side effects than synthetic progestins.

Natural progesterone is available by a doctor's prescription from a compounding pharmacy. (It can also be found in some—but not all—of the progesterone creams sold in health food stores, but you may have to do some checking to make sure it's present in significant amounts—at least 400 milligrams per ounce of cream.) You should work with a practitioner to arrange a cyclical progesterone schedule, suggests Dr. Hudson. "There are lots of different ways to do it, depending on the problem."

Try the cream or oral micronized forms of progesterone first, recommends Dr. Hudson. If they don't work to control bleeding, she'll try Micronor, a synthetic progestin she finds her patients tolerate better than Provera.

Herbs. Dr. Hudson also uses herbs with a progesterone-like effect, such as chasteberry. "It's the number one herb to manage chronic abnormal bleeding. You have to try it for three to four months to see if it has an effect," she says. She suggests women try a 40-milligram capsule of standardized extract or 40 drops of a good quality herbal tincture. But keep in mind that it's not an instant cure for a one-time heavy period.

Other herbs women have tried and found beneficial include trillium, cotton, cinnamon oil tincture, and ergot. Because they are so potent, they can't be obtained over the counter—they must come from a practitioner. "They have to be used in really specific doses, so it's not a do-it-yourself thing," Dr. Hudson says. More readily available herbs to manage heavy bleeding include ginger, yarrow, and shepherd's purse. Often, she combines herbs with natural progesterone and nutrients such as vitamin C and bioflavonoids. "For bleeding, the treatment plan can be fairly complex."

Endometriosis. Some scientists are looking into the possibility of an immune dysfunction contributing to endometriosis, notes Dr. Hudson. She uses herbs that power the immune response, such as echinacea, pokeroot, and astragalus. "Some that I use, like aconite, bryonia, and gelsemium, can't be self-prescribed. Their purpose is to aid the immune response, and these three herbs can be toxic if dosed incorrectly."

The treatment program is often very complicated, says Dr. Hudson. "But I would say that most—but not all—cases of endometriosis respond to a natural approach." She suggests that women find a naturopath since they are trained in many modalities including herbs and nutrition.

Tess Thompson, of the Endometriosis Association, adds that many of her organization's members have given positive feedback on their experiences with acupuncture, homeopathy, and better nutrition. (Information on alternative approaches is available from the association.)

For the pain of endometriosis, Dr. Hudson uses antispasmodic herbs like viburnum, belladonna, and cimicifuga.

"There is some evidence that chiropractic might be helpful for painful periods," adds Dr. Fugh-Berman.

Fibroids. "I wouldn't let women get overly optimistic that natural medicine will cure their fibroids," says Dr. Hudson. "This is the gynecological condition that I most often end up having to refer back to a medical doctor for surgery. In my experience, nothing in alternative medicine consistently and reliably shrinks fibroids."

Among the measures that haven't worked for the majority of her patients: hot castor oil compresses, strict dairy- and meat-free low-fat diets, high soy diets, Traditional Chinese Medicine, natural progesterone, hormone balancing treatments, and liver detoxification. Dr. Fugh-Berman concurs, "Even practitioners of Chinese Medicine tell me that it works better for small fibroids than large ones—and small fibroids aren't usually a problem."

So, says Dr. Hudson, "My approach to fibroids is to see if we can manage the symptoms, such as bleeding and cramping, until the woman becomes menopausal. At that time, fibroids tend to shrink since there is less estrogen to stimulate them."

part two

Disease-Free

2

Quick Quiz

How Healthy Is Your Family Tree?

Both your mother and your father can pass on to you a genetic predisposition to certain health problems. But experts are now noticing an especially strong mother-daughter link. Just because your mom had, say, breast cancer doesn't mean that you're going to develop it, however. In general, the more close relatives you have with a condition, and the younger they were when they developed it, the more susceptible you are to it.

What does your mother's health mean for you? To find out, first answer the following 10 questions. Then for each yes response, read the corresponding explanation below.

____1. Has your mom had breast cancer?

____2. Has your mom had heart trouble?

____3. Is your mom overweight?

____4. Does your mom have Type II (adult-onset) diabetes?

____5. Does your mom have fibroids?

____6. Were your mom's pregnancies especially difficult?

____7. When did your mom go through menopause?

____8. Does your mom have osteoporosis?

____9. Has your mom experienced a major depressive illness?

___10. Does your mom abuse alcohol?

What Your Yes Means

1. "Fewer than 10 percent of all breast cancers are hereditary," says Henry T. Lynch, M.D., president of the Hereditary Cancer Institute in Omaha, Nebraska. "But having a mother or sister with breast cancer puts you at a two to three times greater risk of inheriting this disease."

What you can do: Eat low-fat, high-fiber foods; exercise regularly; cut back on alcohol; and quit smoking. Also consider getting a mammogram every year or so as early as age 30 rather than at 40 or 50. Certainly do a monthly breast self-exam. (For more information about prevention and early detection, see Breakthroughs in Breast Health on page 47.)

2. If your mother had a heart attack before age 65, heart trouble may very well be in your future. What's more, you can inherit certain risk factors, such as high cholesterol and high blood pressure, that can make you more susceptible to heart problems, says Jan Breslow, M.D., an expert in

genetics and professor at Rockefeller University in New York City.

What you can do: Stay slim, exercise regularly, refrain from smoking, and cut back on fatty foods. Also, have your blood pressure and cholesterol levels checked regularly. (For more information on preventing and treating heart problems, see What You Need to Know about Heart Disease on page 55.)

3. "Some women are simply predisposed to being heavy," says Claude Bouchard, Ph.D., professor of exercise physiology at Laval University in Quebec City, Canada. "Research has shown that body weight is 25 to 40 percent hereditary."

But some genes may affect your figure more than others. One landmark study of 540 people found that a woman's weight correlates more with her mother's size than with her father's. So if your mom is 20 to 30 pounds overweight, you have a two to three times greater chance of putting on that much weight, too. If she is obese, your risk of obesity may increase as much as sixfold.

What you can do: Go easy on fats and sweets and exercise regularly. (For more specific strategies, turn to part 3.)

4. Type II diabetes—which tends to occur after age 40—is very common in women. It also seems to be passed along more easily by mothers than by fathers, says Mayer B. Davidson, M.D., president of the American Diabetes Association. In fact, studies show that if your mother has Type II diabetes, you're 20 to 40 percent more likely to develop the condition than if your father has it.

What you can do: Stay slim and exercise regularly. A diabetes test is recommended once every three years after age 45. But if your mother has diabetes, get screened at a younger age and on a more frequent basis. Your doctor can advise you.

5. Although one out of four women of childbearing age have uterine fibroids, these benign growths seem to cluster in some families more than in others. Some scientists even suspect that women whose female relatives had problems with fibroids (such as heavy menstrual bleeding) are more prone to them as well. "We're now trying to confirm this by surveying women who've had problematic fibroids to find out whether fibroid trouble runs in their families," says Cynthia Morton, Ph.D., professor of obstetrics and gynecology at Harvard Medical School.

What you can do: If your fibroids are causing abnormal uterine bleeding, your doctor may prescribe oral contraceptives. The growths can also be surgically removed.

6. If you've not yet had children, your mother's experience during pregnancy can give you a clue as to what to expect, says Robert J. Sokol, M.D., dean of Wayne State University School of Medicine in Detroit. For instance, there may be similarities in the size and shape of your pelvis or

(continued)

in how your uterus contracts, which can influence whether or not your delivery will be easy. Some families tend to bear babies way past their due dates. Further, research has shown that high blood pressure and varicose veins in pregnancy also run in families.

What you can do: Get prenatal care to reduce your risk of complications. As for varicose veins, the best way to minimize them is to maintain a healthy weight and wear support stockings during your pregnancy. As a last resort, varicose veins can be surgically removed post-pregnancy.

7. "You're very likely to reach menopause at the same age your mother did," says Wulf H. Utian, M.D., Ph.D., executive director of the North American Menopause Society. "There's something in the genetic process that determines how many eggs a woman has at birth and influences how fast she loses them over the next 50 years or so."

What you can do: If you smoke, quit. Cigarettes can cause menopause to happen two to three years early. (For the latest information on hormone replacement therapy during menopause, see Hormone Replacement Update on page 26.)

8. "The amount of bone a woman has, and the rate at which she loses it, will closely resemble that of her mother," says Felicia Cosman, M.D., clinical director of the National Osteoporosis Foundation. Research has shown that the daughters of women with osteoporosis have a higher incidence of brittle bones. As a result, they're more likely to have backaches, hip fractures, and a stooped posture.

What you can do: Increase your intake of calcium and vitamin D, either from food or supplements. Strength-training exercises, cutting back on alcohol, and not smoking also keep bones strong. (For more skeleton-saving advice, see The Latest Strategies for Stronger Bones on page 64.)

9. "A woman has a 10 percent chance of inheriting her mother's mood disorders," says Shari I. Lusskin, M.D., assistant professor of psychiatry at New York University Medical Center in New York City. "So if your mother experienced postpartum depression, you're more likely to become depressed after giving birth."

What you can do: Watch for any warning signs of depression, such as crying spells and sudden mood swings. If you suspect a problem, consult a mental health professional.

10. Alcoholism runs in families, says Artemis P. Simopoulos, M.D., president of the Center for Genetics, Nutrition, and Health in Washington, D.C. Women are especially vulnerable: Research has shown that the daughters of women with drinking problems are three times more likely to become alcoholic than the daughters of men with drinking problems.

What you can do: If your drinking interferes with your responsibilities, or if loved ones hint that you have a problem, seek treatment.

Breakthroughs in Breast Health

From examinations to nutritional changes to chemotherapy, the war against breast cancer is being waged on many fronts. The good news is that breast cancer can be treated successfully when it is caught early. Enlist the strategies below in your battle for breast health.

Know Thyself

Performing breast self examination (BSE) on a monthly basis gives you the opportunity to become familiar with how your breasts look and feel. A woman who regularly performs BSE is more likely to find an abnormality at an earlier, treatable stage because she knows the contours of her breasts so well.

At least one recent large-scale study, which tracked more than 250,000 women for 5 years, suggested that women who perform regular BSE fail to find any more cancers than women who don't. But even the study's authors admit that they need to look at 7 to 10 years' worth of data before knowing for certain whether or not BSE is of benefit.

In the meantime, many doctors agree that BSE should not be abandoned. "In the absence of randomized, controlled trials—which are very expensive and hard to do—medicine is based on experience," notes Daniel B. Kopans, M.D., a leading authority in breast cancer detection, associate professor of radiology at

Tamoxifen Cuts Breast Cancer Rate

Early detection and treatment have long been a woman's only "protection" against breast cancer. Now, for the first time in history, a prescription drug called tamoxifen (Nolvadex) offers hope for preventing the disease in the first place.

Tamoxifen is not a new drug. Doctors have been using it for 20 years as a treatment for breast cancer. But researchers from the National Surgical Adjuvant Breast and Bowel Project in Pittsburgh—with support from the National Cancer Institute—decided to study whether tamoxifen could actually thwart breast cancer in women at high risk for the disease.

For their groundbreaking Breast Cancer Prevention Trial, the researchers followed 13,388 women at high risk for breast cancer. The women were divided into two groups. One group was given tamoxifen; the other was given a placebo (a fake pill). Data gathered six years into the study showed that tamoxifen cut the incidence of breast cancer by 45 percent. The researchers were so pleased with the findings that they halted the trial and announced their findings 14 months ahead of schedule.

Taking tamoxifen is not without risk, however. According to the early results of the trial, the drug did increase the women's chances of three rare but life-threatening health problems. Thirty-three members of the tamoxifen group developed endometrial cancer (cancer of the lining of the uterus), compared with 14 members of the placebo group. Seventeen tamoxifen-takers experienced pulmonary embolism (blood clot in the lung), compared with 6 placebo-takers. And 30 of the tamoxifen-takers developed deep-vein thrombosis (blood clots in major veins), compared with 19 of the placebo-takers.

Whether or not to take tamoxifen is a highly individual decision. The benefits must be weighed against the risks, taking into account a woman's age, personal health history, and family health history. If you are at high risk for breast cancer, ask your doctor if tamoxifen is the right choice for you.

HEALTH FLASH

Harvard Medical School, and director of breast imaging at Massachusetts General Hospital in Boston. "And experience is that you can find small cancers by breast self-examination."

To learn how to perform a thorough self-exam, ask your physician, contact your local office of the American Cancer Society, or call a local hospital or health clinic.

Ease Mammogram Anxiety

Women are inundated with news about breast cancer and the importance of getting mammograms regularly. So why are so many of us reluctant to be screened?

"What we have in the media is lots of talk about how prevalent breast cancer is," says Elizabeth A. Patterson, M.D., assistant professor of radiology and a breast imager at the University of Pennsylvania Medical Center in Philadelphia. "What we don't have is much information on how successfully we can treat it when we catch it early with mammography."

Here are the three main reasons women give for not getting mammograms, and how to overcome them and go for a screening.

Something might show up. There are some things you simply don't want to know. Your new assistant's politics, your teenage son's diet during the school day—in essence, stuff that's worrisome but utterly out of your control. By this definition, the possibility that you might have breast cancer doesn't qualify, but not everyone knows it.

"There are still some women who believe very strongly that breast cancer is a death sentence," says Dr. Patterson. They don't want to know about it because they believe there's nothing they can do about it.

In two words: They're wrong. Yes, breast cancer is scary. It's the most prevalent type of cancer in women, second only to lung cancer in the number of cancer deaths in women per year. "But in the last two years, there's been a very small decline in the percentage of breast cancer deaths; this is a direct result of the impact of mammography," says Carole Chrvala, Ph.D., chief of clinical research for the Food and Drug Administration's (FDA) division of mammography quality and radiation programs. This means you can lick it if you catch it early. And mammography, which can detect a tumor as much as two years before a manual exam, is still the best way we have to do just that.

The solution: "The more proactive women are in selecting their mammography centers and asking questions, the more empowered they'll feel in the process—and in the fight to maintain their health," says Dr. Chrvala.

Begin by calling the National Cancer Institute's Cancer Information Service. You can obtain the 800 number by calling toll-free directory assistance. The service will provide more information on mammograms and a list of accredited, FDA-approved mammography facilities near you. Interview each facility before you settle on a center. Some sample questions: How long does a typical mammogram take? Will I have to wait before I am screened? How

Four Tips for a More Comfortable Mammogram

Getting a mammogram doesn't have to be an unpleasant experience, says John Coscia, M.D., director of clinical breast radiology at the University of Texas Southwestern Medical Center at Dallas. Not every woman finds the procedure uncomfortable, but if you do, his suggestions should make things easier.

1. Schedule your exam during the time in your menstrual cycle when your breasts are the least tender. For most women, this is in the first two weeks after menstruation ends. (According to one study, having a mammogram during this time may also improve accuracy for premenopausal women.)

2. Cut out caffeine, especially coffee, for a week before the exam. "There's good anecdotal evidence that this can help," says Dr. Coscia, though the reason why isn't clear. Taking vitamin E for a few weeks beforehand (400 to 800 international units a day) also seems to help. If you are considering taking amounts above 200 international units, discuss this with your doctor first. One study using low-dose vitamin E supplements showed an increased risk of hemorrhagic stroke.

3. Take an over-the-counter pain reliever about an hour beforehand. Use it afterward, too, if needed.

4. Speak up if you're feeling uncomfortable during the procedure. "The patient should be in control of the exam," says Dr. Coscia. "The breast is compressed against the x-ray plate to improve accuracy, but there's room for adjustment." The technologist giving the exam should be able to make you comfortable without sacrificing the effectiveness of the mammogram.

much does a mammogram cost? Will my insurance cover it completely? How will I be informed of my results? Who will be there to answer my questions?

No one told me to get one. Go to a dentist, and she checks for cavities. She doesn't ask you whether you'd like her to do some oral detective work first, nor do you have to ask her to, well, detect. Detecting's simply what she does. Go to a gynecologist, however, and the care you receive isn't always up to code—at least when it comes to mammograms.

"Mammography is one of the only medical areas that requires you to be proactive," explains Dr. Chrvala. "Your physician doesn't ask you if you want a breast check or Pap test when you go in for your yearly exam. And she doesn't rely on you to bring it up. She just goes ahead and does both. But mammograms are different."

Mammograms are prescribed, not perfunctory. And many women feel their doctors don't prescribe them. "Women typically say that their doctors don't give them the message that they need regular mammograms," says Dr. Chrvala. And doctors? "They typically say they do." What this means, says Dr. Chrvala, is that doctors probably aren't encouraging their patients to get mammograms in a way that's compelling to women. For instance, they might say, "It's time for you to think about having a mammogram," instead of, "You need to get a mammogram. Now."

The solution: "My best advice is to find a gynecologist you can team up with," says Kathryn Kash, Ph.D., director of psychosocial services at the Strang-Cornell Cancer Prevention Center in New York City. "I'm talking about a physician who'll really listen to your concerns. Look for someone who won't simply recommend that you have regular mammograms, but a doctor who either suggests a facility and has her assistant make the appointment for you, or someone who won't skip a beat if you ask for that much."

I'm not at risk. Most women know that breast cancer strikes one in eight women, but they're not convinced that they themselves are at any risk for the disease. So they don't get screened. "I've done research that indicates that women aren't always able to correctly identify the risk factors for breast cancer, yet they often decide for themselves that they're not at risk," points out Dr. Chrvala.

This seems reasonable, really, when you consider that doctors aren't even sure what causes breast cancer. Here's what they do know: The primary risk factors (those that double your risk) include a family history of the disease (meaning you have a first-degree relative—mother, sister, or daughter—who has had breast cancer), a personal history of breast cancer, and a personal history of previous biopsies that revealed cellular changes (*atypical hyperplasia* in med-speak) in your breasts.

That's it for the biggies. Other more minor risk factors (those that boost your risk by about 20 percent) include never having children, having your first child after age 30, getting your period before you're 12 years old, and starting menopause after age 50, all of which expose you to more menstrual periods and, therefore, more of the hormonal changes that doctors speculate are behind some breast cancers. In addition, there's what Dr. Chrvala deems fairly convincing evidence that women who eat a high-fat, low-fiber diet; drink the equivalent of more than two glasses of wine a day; and don't exercise regularly are at greater risk for breast cancer.

That said, however, Dr. Chrvala points out that a full 75 percent of women who are diagnosed with the disease don't have any of the risk factors. This means that all women are at some risk. "Simply being a woman puts you there," sums up Dr. Chrvala.

The solution: Discuss your chances of developing breast cancer with your physician and plan to minimize your risk by eating a low-fat, high-fiber diet; exercising regularly; drinking no more than two glasses of wine a day; not smoking; examining your breasts once a month, the same time every month, noting any changes you feel; and—you got it—having regular mammograms.

A Simple Saliva Test

Doctors may one day be able to diagnose breast cancer simply by asking patients to spit into a cup. In a study of 28 patients, researchers at the University of Mississippi Medical Center in Jackson recently isolated a substance in saliva that appears to be a marker for breast cancer. If confirmed in a larger study, these results could eventually lead to a home test for breast cancer. "We're currently studying whether there are markers for oral cancer and prostate cancer as well," says Charles Streckfus, D.D.S., lead researcher and professor of diagnostic sciences.

Get Moving

Does exercising reduce breast cancer risk? One of the biggest investigations done on the topic suggests that the answer is yes. Researchers in Norway traced the health of more than 25,000 women over a nine-year period. They found that women who exercised at least four hours a week had a 37 percent lower breast cancer risk, compared with women who did no exercise at all. They also found that women who were very active at work—those whose jobs involved lots of lifting and walking—reduced their risk by about one-fourth.

Does this mean you should run out and get a job delivering pianos? That would be premature (and a bad career move). But taking the stairs instead of the elevator, using the copier down the hall, and otherwise being more active in your day-to-day life could help. "We're not sure how much exercise women need to do," says Anne McTiernan, M.D., Ph.D., of the Fred Hutchinson Cancer Research Center in Seattle. "But we do know that women who are overweight have an increased risk of breast cancer."

Of course, says Dr. McTiernan, "The more exercise you do, the better." That's for a whole host of reasons, ranging from lower blood pressure to reduced risk of diabetes. Breast cancer risk hasn't been definitively added to that list . . . yet. But exercise now, and odds are you won't regret it later. (Of course, be careful not to overdo.)

Fight Back with Food

Put these foods on your grocery list. Recent studies have linked each one to fighting breast cancer.

❖ Orange and grapefruit juices. Researchers at the University of Western Ontario in London, Canada, gave mice either double-strength orange or grapefruit juice or plain drinking water.

After the mice were injected with human breast-cancer cells, the juice groups got 50 percent fewer tumors, and the tumors were 50 percent less likely to spread. What did it? Two special compounds, hesperidin in oranges and naringin in grapefruit, may be partly responsible, researchers say. Keep in mind that what works in animals doesn't always work in people—we'll need more studies to find that out.

❖ Wheat bran cereal. Women who ate a daily half-cup serving of All-Bran— enough to deliver 10 grams of fiber from wheat bran—saw drops in their estrogen levels. Experts think that high levels of estrogen stimulate breast cancer.

❖ Canola oil. This vegetable oil is rich in an omega-3 fatty acid. A study at the University of California, Los Angeles, is now testing whether omega-3's can prevent recurrence of cancer in breast cancer survivors, partly because women from countries with less breast cancer have higher tissue levels of omega-3's. Other top sources include salmon and white (albacore) tuna.

❖ Soy milk. Women in Australia who excreted the most isoflavones, a compound found in soy milk and other soy foods, were 73 percent less likely to have breast cancer than women who excreted the least.

❖ Carrots and spinach. Compared with women who ate carrots or spinach more than twice a week, women who never ate them had twice the risk of breast cancer.

❖ Yogurt. In a test-tube study, yogurt slowed the growth of breast cancer

Heat-Seeking Pads May Find Breast Cancer Sooner

Heat-sensitive pads that you slip into your bra at the doctor's office may be a new way to detect breast diseases, including cancer. Unlike mammograms, the pads produce no radiation exposure, and they're effective on the dense breast tissue of younger women. They rely on the fact that cancer cells have a more active metabolism than normal cells and so generate more heat. After they're worn for 15 minutes during a doctor visit, pads from both breasts are compared for temperature differences. "If any are found, it means the breast needs to be examined more carefully," explains Everett M. Lautin, M.D., a diagnostic radiologist at Albert Einstein College of Medicine/Montefiore Medical Center in New York City.

The pads have been cleared for use as an addition to standard screening and are being marketed as the BreastAlert Differential Temperature Sensor by HumaScan, which is located in Cranford, New Jersey. They may prove most useful to women under 40, who don't usually have mammograms unless a suspicious lump is detected by physical examination, Dr. Lautin says. The pads may be able to detect breast changes much earlier than a physical exam, although it's not certain yet whether they can detect breast diseases earlier than mammograms can, he explains. The pads might also be used in older women between mammograms.

cells, even if the yogurt's active bacterial cultures were removed first. This hints that any yogurt—not just the kind with live and active cultures—may be protective, for reasons yet unknown.

Don't Shun the Sun

Researchers who studied health data on nearly 5,000 women found that breast cancer risk in women who reported getting the most sun exposure was about 30 to 40 percent lower than the risk among women who got the least sun. A similar reduction in risk was found among women who lived in sunny climes.

The key to this phenomenon may be vitamin D, which is produced in our skin when it's exposed to sunlight. It only takes about 10 to 15 minutes of sun exposure a day to get the vitamin D your body needs, says the study's author, Esther John, Ph.D., an epidemiologist at the Northern California Cancer Center in Union City. "And that's just casual exposure—the sunlight you get on your face and neck and arms and hands when you're regularly dressed," she explains. So while the exact dose of sunlight needed is unknown, taking a brief outdoor stroll (without sunscreen) seems a prudent way to try to benefit from the sun's cancer-fighting power. (Prolonged, unprotected exposure to sunlight is to be avoided since it raises your risk of skin cancer.)

Getting vitamin D in your diet (primarily from milk) and from supplements may also help, says Dr. John. This is especially true if you live in northern latitudes, where taking a multivitamin with 400 international units (IU), the current Daily Value, may be beneficial. (Just don't try for too much vitamin D. Levels well above 2,000 IU on a regular basis can be harmful.)

What You Need to Know about Heart Disease

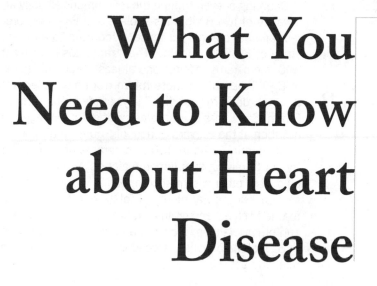

Heart disease is the number one killer of women, yet it's misdiagnosed with frightening regularity. Just ask Nancy Beall, a 57-year-old administrative assistant from Baltimore. She had a heart attack in 1996 and didn't know it. "I sat up all night long," says Beall. "It was like all the muscles in my body felt tired and weak. All my joints hurt. I thought, 'Gosh, maybe I have rheumatoid arthritis!' I had achiness in my arms. But there was nothing that I would call pain."

Early in the morning, she called the cardiologist who had been caring for her for years. "He just happened to be in his office at 7:00 A.M., standing by the phone. He told me to go straight to the emergency room. He ordered me to tell the attending doctor that I have atypical symptoms and to consult with him while waiting for the results."

Beall called an ambulance immediately and went to the hospital. The emergency room doctors did two cardiac enzyme tests, which showed no sign of a heart attack. They told her she had a flu and wanted to send her home. "But my daughter kept insisting that they do the test again—she kept repeating that my symptoms were 'atypical.'" Sure enough, the third enzyme test showed that she had really had a heart attack.

"It turned out that three of my four heart arteries were 99 percent obstructed," Beall says. Her life was saved by an immediate quadruple bypass.

Two B or Not Two B

Doubling or even tripling the recommended daily allowance of two B vitamins—folate and B_6—may protect against coronary disease, according to a recent study of 80,000 women. (That translates to at least 360 micrograms of folate and at least three milligrams of B_6.) "You absorb more folate from a supplement than you do from your diet," says study author Eric B. Rimm, Sc.D., assistant professor of epidemiology and nutrition at the Harvard School of Public Health. Most multivitamins contain 400 micrograms of folate. But try not to rely on supplements alone. "You'll miss out on a lot of other essential compounds found in foods," says Dr. Rimm. Eat plenty of folate-rich foods like B-fortified cereals and grains, orange juice, kidney beans and other legumes, broccoli, and spinach. Foods rich in B_6 include bananas, avocados, lean chicken, brown rice, and oats.

Like the emergency room doctors, many people still think of heart attacks as a man's problem. The truth is that heart disease kills more women every year than all forms of cancer, chronic lung disease, pneumonia, diabetes, accidents, and AIDS combined. That's more than a half-million women.

And it's not just women who underestimate their risk. Even some doctors still think of heart disease as primarily a man's problem. Studies have found that doctors provide women with less testing, less follow-up, less treatment, and less surgery.

That may partly explain why, once heart disease does strike, it's far deadlier for women. Women are more than 1½ times as likely to die within a year of their first heart attack than are men.

Here is what you need to know about the symptoms of a heart attack, what new testing devices are available, an important new link between heart disease and depression, and the risk factors for heart disease that you should consider.

Women's Symptoms: Different, but Just As Deadly

What does a heart attack feel like? For men, it's often the classic chest-clutching pain, tightness, or heaviness in the chest, usually accompanied by shortness of breath or sweating.

For women, a heart attack can be completely different. Women may experience little or no chest pain, says cardiologist Roy Ziegelstein, M.D., deputy chairman of the department of medicine at the Johns Hopkins Bayview Medical Center in Baltimore. Because the symptoms may be so unlike a typical male heart attack, female symptoms may be described as atypical.

During a heart attack, women often experience shortness of breath or difficulty breathing and may even have pain or weakness in their shoulders, arms, or all over their bodies. Women are more likely than men to experience what feels like nausea, which is not relieved by antacids or burping. There may even be vomiting. The symptoms are more likely to occur when they're resting, or during mental stress or physical exercise. Women are also likely to experience fatigue. "Not, I-fall-asleep-at-5:00-P.M.-every-night fatigue," Dr. Ziegelstein explains, "but feeling completely wiped out." He also cites "a general sense of being unwell—that something really wrong is going on."

In women, atypical symptoms may come and go, signifying angina (a temporary lack of oxygen to the heart, which can be a warning sign of a future heart attack). When they occur at the beginning of a heart attack, symptoms usually don't go away—and they can become worse as minutes or hours pass.

Time Is Muscle: What to Do

Assume that you're having some of these feelings—say, extreme exhaustion, shoulder and arm pain, and fatigue. Something's wrong. Could be flu or a heart attack. How can you tell? "You can't," says Irving Kron, M.D., chief of cardiothoracic surgery at the University of Virginia Medical Center in Charlottesville, and vice-chairman of the American Heart Association Council on Cardiovascular Surgery. "You have something that gets you nervous? Get it checked out."

And do it fast. "Time is muscle," says D. Douglas Miller, M.D., professor of internal medicine and medical director of the Cardiac Stress Laboratory at St. Louis University. Don't delay. Here's what to do.

1. Call your doctor. If you can't reach your doctor, make sure you let the person on the other end know that you believe it's a medical emergency.
2. Take an aspirin. "Chewing a 325-milligram aspirin in the early stages of a heart attack has been shown to improve the rate of survival in men and women," says Dr. Miller.
3. Head for the emergency room if the symptoms are extreme, and have the medical staff or a family member alert your physician.

Don't worry about your potential embarrassment if you're wrong and really do have the flu. Studies show that women tend to delay much longer than men before showing up at a hospital with a heart attack—as much as four hours longer. "Women and men both have to be willing to feel foolish," says Dr. Kron. "Your chances of surviving, if it is a heart attack, are much better if you're at the hospital than if you're at home wondering."

When describing symptoms to any doctor, be as specific as possible, adds

Marianne Legato, M.D., associate professor of clinical medicine at Columbia University College of Physicians and Surgeons in New York City and author of *The Female Heart.* "Don't say, 'I have a funny feeling.' Say, 'I have chest discomfort when I'm upset. It's a burning pain that goes to my neck and shoulders.'"

Diagnosing Heart Disease

Great technology for diagnosing heart disease in men has been around for a long time. One test is the treadmill stress test, in which an electrocardiogram (EKG) is performed continuously during exercise. This test works fine for men, but in women it produces false positives (indicating that there is a heart problem when there really isn't) more than one-third of the time and false negatives (indicating no problem when there really is one) about one-fourth of the time.

"Women's survival was being harmed," says Dr. Miller. Some women who really didn't have heart disease were sent on for unnecessary and invasive tests. In other cases, some doctors decided to ignore the stress EKG results that showed a problem, betting that the woman was really fine and the machine was wrong. Studies show that after a positive EKG, women are not as likely as men to be given subsequent testing.

Over the past 5 to 10 years, a great deal of effort has been directed toward gender-equivalent testing. "We're now at a point where equivalence is virtually achieved," says Dr. Miller.

The two most accurate new tests involve imaging. "Whenever possible, these are the tests that a woman should ask for," says Rita Redberg, M.D., associate professor of medicine at the University of California, San Francisco, and a member of the American Heart Association Council on Clinical Cardiology.

The first of these new imaging techniques involves having a patient walk on a treadmill, then injecting a radioactive isotope (known as technetium 99 sestamibi) into the bloodstream, which allows special scanners to track the blood flow through the heart. Another option is the stress echocardiogram test. Dr. Legato prefers it because there's no injection, it's accurate, sensitive, and less expensive, and it doesn't take as long as the technetium test.

Not all imaging tests, however, are as good. A far less accurate option is the thallium 201 radioisotope test, which was developed for men but doesn't work as well in women.

Who should get tested? Experts agree that the stress echocardiogram or technetium tests are usually not necessary for premenopausal women who have no risk factors for heart disease.

Women with symptoms or a strong risk factor should get tested, Dr. Legato explains. "I reserve the tests for women who are of some concern for heart disease risk—perhaps they have a new pain, they smoke, they're sedentary, they have a family history of diabetes, or they have diabetes." She recommends testing at least annually for women with symptoms.

If you're going to be tested, Dr. Miller says, it's a good idea to find out what kind of test will be done. If stress EKG or thallium imaging are your only choices, they're better than nothing—but make sure that you follow up with your doctor and ask for retesting if the first test suggests there's a problem.

Depression: Women Must Pay Attention

For both men and women, says Redford Williams, M.D., professor of psychiatry and director of the Behavioral Medicine Research Center at Duke University in Durham, North Carolina, the latest studies link three psychosocial risk factors to a higher risk and worse prognosis for heart disease. They are hostility, social isolation, and depression.

As Dr. Williams explains, men are more likely to have hostility and less likely to have social support. Women tend to have more social support and less hostility—but they're twice as likely to experience depression.

Could depression be one factor explaining why heart disease kills as many women as men? In one study, Nancy Frasure-Smith, Ph.D., associate professor of psychiatry and nursing at Montreal University, tracked 613 men and 283 women who'd had heart attacks. "We found that people who were depressed—men or women—were three to four times more likely to die of cardiac causes. That makes depression as dangerous to the heart as traditional risk factors like high blood pressure or smoking."

To ease the pain, Dr. Legato says, everyone should seek out a confidante, whether it's a doctor, friend, or relative. "Everyone needs someone to whom they can lay out their problems—many times just verbalizing will begin a train of thought that produces a solution."

Reducing Your Risk: What Every Woman Must Know

"The risk factors in women are pretty much the same as they are in men," says John LaRosa, M.D., chancellor of Tulane University Medical Center in New Orleans and a member of the American Heart Association Risk Factors Task Force. "But there are some subtle differences." It's important to know what they are. Here's a review of the major heart disease risk factors—and what you can do about them.

Smoking. Women who smoke heavily increase their heart disease risk two to four times.

What to do: Quit. It works. After smoking cessation, risk in both women and men tumbles within months, and within three to five years is as low as the risk for nonsmokers.

High cholesterol. For men and women with total cholesterol below 150, it is very difficult to get heart disease. When total cholesterol is more than 150, both men and women are more susceptible—and the higher it goes, the more susceptible they are. But important differences between the genders do exist.

Men can generally use their total cholesterol to tell whether they're at risk. But women need to learn their high-density lipoprotein (HDL) and low-density lipoprotein (LDL) numbers. Then, they should divide the total by the HDL. The result is called the total-to-HDL ratio. The goal is to be 4.0 or lower. Anything more than that means an elevated risk of heart disease.

What to do: Exercise regularly and follow a diet that is low in total fat and animal fats to lower bad LDL cholesterol and reduce overall cholesterol. Women under 50 with no risk factors and good readings should have their cholesterol checked every four to five years. Older women or women with less-than-optimal cholesterol levels should have their cholesterol checked annually.

High blood pressure. For both men and women, target blood pressure should be 130 systolic (top), and 85 diastolic (bottom). If either number is higher, it might mean an increased risk of heart disease.

What to do: Have your blood pressure checked at least once a year if you're 40 or younger, twice a year if you're over 40 or you have other risk factors for heart disease. If there's a problem, losing weight, reducing salt, limiting alcohol, and increasing exercise can make a difference. Initial research suggests that for both women and men, treating and controlling hypertension can reduce heart disease risk significantly.

Physical inactivity. Physically active women have a 60 to 75 percent lower risk of heart disease than inactive women. The possible reason for this? Exercise not only improves cholesterol but also may keep blood vessels strong, flexible, and clean.

What to do: Walk two miles a day or the equivalent in another form of exercise. If you haven't exercised in the last year, begin slowly with your doctor's okay.

Diabetes. Regardless of her age, a woman with diabetes has the same risk of heart disease as a man, and a risk three to seven times higher than a woman who doesn't have diabetes.

What to do: Maintain a healthy weight, stay active, and reduce dietary fat intake to help delay and control diabetes. If you do have diabetes, work with your doctor to control heart disease risk factors.

Waist/hip ratio. Both obesity and a high waist/hip ratio are risk factors for heart disease. A high waist/hip ratio usually signifies too much fat on the abdomen. It's a pattern that doctors call central obesity. The pattern is more common among men, but for both genders, it's strongly linked to an increased risk of heart disease—regardless of whether the person is overweight. How can you tell if you have a good waist/hip ratio? Get out the tape measure and measure

Cholesterol: Work the Numbers

If you think you're safe from heart attack because your cholesterol is below 200, think again—you're not really safe until you hit 150 or below.

"If your cholesterol is below 150, you're home free," says William Castelli, M.D., who headed the landmark Framingham (Massachusetts) Heart Study for 16 years. "Virtually no one gets a heart attack at that level. But twice as many people in our country get heart attacks with cholesterol levels between 150 and 200 as those with cholesterol levels over 300. For instance, 35 percent of the people in the Framingham Study who had heart attacks had cholesterol between 150 and 200."

Atherosclerosis—the buildup of plaque in the arteries—starts to accelerate when your cholesterol gets over 150, explains John LaRosa, M.D., chancellor of Tulane University Medical Center in New Orleans and a member of the American Heart Association Risk Factors Task Force. So why does the number 200 stick to our brains like plaque to an artery? "The problem is that we've confused average cholesterol with normal cholesterol," explains Dr. LaRosa. Among Americans today, the average total cholesterol hovers around 215.

But even if your cholesterol is 189 or 198, don't get upset. That one number doesn't tell the whole story. You need to know your high-density lipoprotein (HDL)—the "good" cholesterol—number, too. Then use it to find your total-to-HDL ratio by dividing your total cholesterol number by your HDL number.

If your ratio is 4.0 or lower, you can relax. You're one of the people who really are safe from heart attacks. In fact, some folks with cholesterol over 200 may not have that great a risk because a high HDL can offer protection. But, notes Dr. LaRosa, this HDL protection only goes so far. If your total cholesterol is over 300, it's too high. Here's how to get your HDL number.

Make a date for a profile. Tell your doctor you want to keep tabs on your cholesterol levels and ask her where you can go to get a lipid profile. (Your profile will include your total cholesterol and HDL levels.) If your insurance won't cover it, find a way to pay the $25 to $60. Or call Wal-Mart and find out when a store near you will be offering its $29 lipid profiles. Those tests are accurate, and they'll give you the numbers you need to do the easy math for your ratio.

Get it again. Get at least two cholesterol tests within an eight-week time frame, advises Peter Wilson, M.D., current director of laboratories at the Framingham Heart Study. "There can be a 12-point variation in total cholesterol. And HDL can vary quite a lot, too," he points out. If the difference in cholesterol levels is over 30, take a third test, and then find the average of all three.

Make a note. Whenever you take a cholesterol test—every five years if it's good, every year or more if it's bad—write down the results.

Heart Rx: Lower Your Cholesterol

High cholesterol is one of the easiest problems to control on your own. Here's the basic strategy for lowering your cholesterol and preventing heart disease.

Defat your diet. "If you look at large groups of people, the overwhelming determinant of cholesterol level and cardiac risk is diet and intake of animal fat," says John LaRosa, M.D., chancellor of Tulane University Medical Center in New Orleans and a member of the American Heart Association Risk Factors Task Force. "You just have to get that fat off your plate. That's the key. We are designed to be plant-eaters—we have flat teeth and long intestines for digesting vegetables. We're not meat-eaters, like some bears. They have sharp, tearing teeth, short intestines, and cholesterols of 500, but it's all high-density lipoproteins (HDLs). They never get atherosclerosis because they were meant to eat meat."

A low-fat diet (below 25 percent total fat and below 20 grams in saturated fat) helps lower bad low-density lipoproteins (LDL), so HDL isn't overwhelmed. A diet like this can lower cholesterol 5 to 15 points or more.

While you're eating less meat, eat more fruits and vegetables. The antioxidants in them keep LDL from sticking to the walls of your arteries.

Work it up. Diet and exercise must go together, says William Castelli, M.D., who headed the landmark Framingham (Massachusetts) Heart Study for 16 years. The beauty of this combo is that exercise raises your HDL levels while the diet lowers your LDL.

And each milligram per deciliter of HDL in your blood has three times the impact of one milligram per deciliter of total cholesterol, says Peter Wilson, M.D., current director of laboratories at the Framingham Heart Study. "If I had to choose, I'd rather my HDL went up five milligrams per deciliter than my total cholesterol went down five," he says.

There's some controversy about the level of exercise intensity you should aim for. The best data come from runners, experts say. One study from Georgetown University in Washington, D.C., found that of 2,906 people, those who jogged between 11 and 14 miles a week had levels of HDL 11 percent higher than those who didn't exercise. If jogging's not for you, follow Dr. Castelli's prescription—a 2-mile (or more) walk every day. "Distance counts," he says. If diet and exercise aren't enough to score a ratio below 4.0 after four months, you may need cholesterol-lowering medications. But even if you do, you probably won't need to take quite as much.

the number of inches around your waist. Then measure your hips at the widest part. Now simply divide the waist measure by the hip measure to get the ratio. The target is 0.8 or below. Above 0.8, research shows that the risk of heart disease rises steeply in women.

What to do: Lose some weight. The good news is that it's not so hard to change a waist/hip ratio by losing a little weight. Even five pounds can make the difference.

High triglycerides. High triglycerides are more powerful predictors of risk in women than men, especially after women reach age 50. "Triglycerides are not cholesterol, but they're a marker for the same carriers that bring cholesterol to the blood vessel wall," explains Dr. LaRosa. "Anything more than 150 begins to accelerate the uptake of cholesterol into the blood vessel wall. The 200 to 400 range is borderline—there may be some increased risk. More than 400, everyone agrees, is too high." Triglycerides are usually measured as part of a routine cholesterol screening. Ask your doctor about it.

What to do: Weight loss—even as little as 15 pounds around the waist—can reduce triglycerides.

Age. Men's risk of heart attack and stroke soars after age 45. In women, the risk rises when they're about 10 years older. Researchers believe that the gradual drop in estrogen after menopause may be partly responsible. Women well past menopause, especially over 60, are at the greatest risk for heart attack. Past age 60, one in four women as well as one in four men will die of heart disease.

In premenopausal women without any major risk factors, the risk of coronary disease is pretty low. (The exception to this is if the woman smokes and takes oral contraceptives together, says Dr. LaRosa. "They increase their risk of coronary disease about 30-fold.") A postmenopausal woman's risk for a coronary event is four times the risk of a premenopausal woman of the same age. But don't feel invincible if you're premenopausal. The disease processes that lead to heart disease start young. Regardless of your age, the sooner you start with prevention and detection, the better.

What to do: While there's not much you can do about your age, there is research suggesting that estrogen replacement therapy (ERT) can significantly reduce postmenopausal women's heart disease risk. It may reduce LDL and increase HDL by 10 to 15 percent. Of course, there is controversy over the use of ERT, and it's a complex decision that women must make with their doctors. Minimizing all the other risk factors that you have control over—like diet and exercise—can make a big difference.

Family history and race. A family history of heart disease is even more common in women with coronary heart disease than men. Your risk of heart disease is higher if a close member had the disease. Race makes a difference, too: African-Americans have a higher risk than Caucasians, partly because of a tendency toward high blood pressure.

What to do: Adopt heart-healthy habits and get regular and complete checkups. African-Americans and anyone with a family history of heart disease should be particularly vigilant.

The Latest Strategies for Stronger Bones

M ost of us know that osteoporosis is a debilitating disease that strikes older women (one in two women over 50 will get it). But many of us don't know that there are simple lifestyle changes we can make in our twenties, thirties, and forties to help keep our skeletons strong for a lifetime, says Ethel Siris, M.D., director of the osteoporosis program at Columbia-Presbyterian Medical Center in New York City. And an anti-osteoporosis program of regular exercise and calcium-rich foods will tone and trim your body right now.

Osteoporosis is a disease characterized by thin, fragile bones—in particular, of the hip, spine, and wrist—that can fracture on the slightest impact. According to experts, 10 million Americans, most of them women, have the disease. Osteoporosis is so common that a woman's lifetime risk of fracturing her hip is equal to her risk of breast, ovarian, and uterine cancers combined.

Bone Basics

Bone is composed of calcium and other minerals. The strength of our bones is in their thickness—called bone mass or density—which peaks when we are between the ages of 20 and 30. If you were to peer through a powerful microscope inside the bone of a 25-year-old woman, you'd see that the building and repair process is constant. Cells called osteoclasts tear down (or resorb) old bone, and cells called osteoblasts build new bone. Until we reach age 25, more bone is formed than is resorbed. Once we've reached our maximum bone density between 25 and 30, bone formation and resorption are basically balanced. But at menopause, the drop in estrogen causes the osteoclasts to rev up their activity. The result is bone loss, explains Sydney Lou Bonnick, M.D., author of *The Osteoporosis Handbook*.

To some degree, our peak bone density is determined by our genes, just like our weight, says Bess Dawson-Hughes, M.D., professor of medicine and chief of the calcium and bone metabolism laboratory at the USDA Human Nutrition Research Center at Tufts University in Medford, Massachusetts. For example, Caucasian and Asian women are more prone to osteoporosis than African-American women. But all women can help influence bone mass via exercise and good nutrition.

During the first five years after menopause, when estrogen drops dramatically, women can lose up to 15 percent of their bone mass, with lesser losses afterward. For a small number of women, thin, fragile bones have been pretty much determined by their genes or medical problems, and rapid, immediate postmenopausal loss will set them on the road to osteoporosis unless drug therapies intervene (see "The Latest on Drug Therapy" on page 72). For many women, however, that 15 percent reduction in bone mass is not significant because they built enough skeletal strength and thickness in their youth through diet and exercise.

Bone-Saving Strategies for Every Age

Here's what you can do to decrease your chances of developing osteoporosis.

20 to 30 years old. In these years, you build more bone than you lose, reaching peak density between 25 and 30. Since your bone mass begins declining after 30, it's essential that you build as much strength as possible now—so your body has a large bone "reserve" to keep your skeleton strong and straight in the future.

What to do: Get 1,000 milligrams of calcium and 200 international units (IU) of vitamin D every day. And do weight-bearing exercises regularly. Avoid fad diets, smoking, having more than two alcoholic drinks a day, and excess salt intake; they can all contribute to bone loss. If your periods are noticeably very irregular (usually the result of hormonal factors, overstrenuous exercising, or anorexia), you could be at higher risk for osteoporosis because estrogen encourages bone strength. Talk to your doctor about the possibility of taking oral contraceptives that contain estrogen.

31 to 50 years old. During these two decades, you may begin to lose a little bone mass—approximately ½ percent a year.

What to do: Keep working that body and eating a bone-building diet; you still need 1,000 milligrams of calcium and 200 IU of vitamin D daily. If you have any risk factors, as described in "Are You at Risk?" talk to your physician about the possibility of getting a bone-density test now. Osteoporosis is often called the silent disease because it can take years for symptoms to appear.

51 to 55 years old (or the five years after menopause). You can lose up to 15 percent of your bone mass in this five-year period.

What to do: This is the prime time for preventive measures. Get a bone-density test now. Continue to combat loss of bone mass with resistance training and weight-bearing exercise (that is, any activity in which you work against gravity). Studies show that exercise can preserve and even build bone in postmenopausal women. And up your calcium intake to 1,200 to 1,500 milligrams (unless you're on estrogen, in which case 1,000 to 1,200 milligrams is fine), while increasing your vitamin D intake to 400 IU. If you're at high risk for osteoporosis or have the disease, talk to your doctor about the possibility of taking an anti-osteoporosis drug. You should also consult a bone specialist for a customized exercise program that safely strengthens your bones. Finally, make your home "fallproof." The National Osteoporosis Foundation has excellent tips on this; write to them at National Osteoporosis Foundation, Department MQ, P.O. Box 96616, Washington, D.C. 20077-7456.

56 to 70 years old. Bone loss slows to about 1 percent a year.

What to do: Keep working out. Make sure your diet includes 1,200 to 1,500 milligrams of calcium and 600 IU of vitamin D; one study showed that a daily regimen of calcium and vitamin D reduced the risk of hip fractures by almost a

Are You at Risk?

Talk to your doctor about the possibility of bone-density testing if one or more of the statements below is true for you.

1. You're premenopausal and your period has stopped for six months or more (not because of pregnancy), which means there's less bone-building estrogen in your body. This is most often the result of overstrenuous exercise or extreme dieting. Thyroid disease, emotional stress, or a pituitary tumor can occasionally be the cause.
2. As an adult, you've broken a bone from a minimal impact injury (for example, you break a rib during a coughing fit, as opposed to in a car accident).
3. You have a strong family history of osteoporosis.
4. You have taken glucocorticoid or some other anti-seizure medications for a long period, or you have overused thyroid medication.
5. You have hyperthyroidism or hyperparathyroidism, both of which interfere with your body's ability to absorb calcium, and thus increase the rate of bone loss.
6. You had a hysterectomy before menopause, with removal of the ovaries (oophorectomy) and without estrogen replacement therapy.
7. You were laid up in bed for six months or longer as an adult.
8. You have more than two alcoholic drinks a day.
9. You smoke.
10. You have a sedentary lifestyle and eat a diet that's low in calcium and vitamin D.
11. You're underweight (so there's less weight loading, which builds bone).

third in postmenopausal women. If you discover that you have osteoporosis, it's not too late to reap benefits from calcium and vitamin D, estrogen or another bone-preserving drug, and specially prescribed, safe exercises.

The Exercise Prescription

Besides reducing the risk of heart disease, adult-onset diabetes, and certain cancers—as well as easing stress—regular exercise is essential for preventing osteoporosis.

Be sure to do a weight-bearing workout—walking, jogging, hiking, stair-climbing, jumping rope—at least three times a week for a minimum of 30 minutes. This type of exercise is a must for maintaining and building bone strength. Just look at what happened to the early astronauts: After three months of weightlessness in space, they lost 10 to 15 percent of their bone density. (Swimming and bicycling, while good for the heart and other muscles, don't much help bones.)

Haven't exercised in a while? Walk slowly for 20 minutes, three times a week, until you feel comfortable with a brisk pace, recommends Barbara Drinkwater, Ph.D., a research physiologist in the department of medicine at the Pacific Medical Center in Seattle, and one of the country's preeminent exercise specialists. If you're already walking briskly for 20 minutes, three or four times a week, increase gradually to an hour at a time.

If you're on a supertight schedule, try fitting in two 15-minute walks when you don't have time for a half-hour stroll; take the stairs instead of the elevator; park far away from your office; and go to the gym instead of having lunch with a friend.

In addition to walking, dancing, and other weight-bearing exercises, it's important to do resistance training (free weights or Nautilus) at least twice a week for 40 minutes. A study conducted by Miriam Nelson, Ph.D., at Tufts University showed that just two 40-minute sessions of resistance training per week for a year allowed postmenopausal women to not only maintain bone mass but also increase it by 1 percent. Do resistance training a maximum of two or three times a week, with at least a day's rest in between, advises Dr. Nelson.

Look for weight-bearing opportunities in daily life, too: Every time there's a choice between carrying the groceries a few blocks or dumping them in the car, carry them, says Dr. Drinkwater. When you're out for a walk, choose a route that has hills. Any chance you have in the course of your everyday life to lift, push, or shove—done carefully, of course, to protect your back—not only exercises your muscles but helps maintain your bone strength as well.

The Calcium Connection

According to government figures, very few American adults consume enough calcium on a daily basis to meet the standards for healthy bones set by the National Institutes of Health. In fact, women older than age 50 average less than half the calcium they need—in part because getting ample calcium through diet alone can be tough. Real tough.

"Some people are either unwilling or unable—often because of low-calorie diets—to eat enough high-calcium foods," says Barbara Levine, R.D., Ph.D., associate clinical professor of nutrition in medicine at Cornell University Medical College in New York City. "For them, a supplement makes real sense."

Consider a recent study of postmenopausal women who added either dry-milk powder or calcium tablets to their daily diets. By the end of the study, both groups had increased their calcium intake. But thanks to the abundance of nutrients in milk, the women eating milk powder had also boosted their intake of zinc, magnesium, potassium, and more, while those taking calcium supplements had not.

But two years after the study ended, the daily calcium intake of the milk-powder group had fallen to about 950 milligrams, while the calcium supplement group was averaging about 1,350 milligrams of calcium a day—not bad, considering their recommended daily intake was 1,500 milligrams.

So for most women, supplements are the most convenient source of calcium. Here are the most common questions concerning calcium—the mineral as well as the supplement—and a guide to getting enough.

How much calcium do I need? According to the National Institutes of Health, women 25 to 49 years of age need 1,000 milligrams of calcium a day, women 50 and older need 1,500 milligrams daily, and pregnant or nursing mothers need 1,200 to 1,500 milligrams a day.

How much calcium should I shoot for in supplements? Here's a quick recommendation some doctors use based on surveys of average calcium intakes nationwide: If your daily requirement is 1,000 milligrams, supplement with 500 milligrams. And if your daily requirement is 1,500 milligrams, supplement with 1,000 milligrams.

For a more tailor-made recommendation, you have to do some homework—but just a smidgen. Simply add up the number of servings you typically eat each day of foods that supply substantial calcium. Most folks, for example, eat at least one of the following single servings daily: eight ounces of nonfat or 1 percent milk, eight ounces of nonfat or low-fat calcium-fortified soy or rice milk, eight ounces of calcium-fortified orange juice, eight ounces of nonfat or low-fat yogurt, and two one-ounce slices of nonfat or reduced-fat cheese.

Once you have a total in mind, multiply that number by 300 for the approximately 300 milligrams of calcium you get per serving of calcium-rich foods. Then add 200 to that sum (for the estimated 200 milligrams of calcium you get from all the other foods you eat throughout the day). Finally, add the milligrams of calcium contained in your multivitamin, if you take one.

The sum total of all your figuring is an estimate of the calcium you consume every day. If that number falls short of your daily requirement, you need to make up the difference, either by eating more calcium-rich foods or by taking a supplement.

Won't my multivitamin give me ample calcium? Unless you get plenty of calcium through your diet, probably not. Most multis have too little calcium to make up for the average shortfall. What they do have, however, is vitamin D, which helps you absorb calcium, and the minerals magnesium, zinc, copper, and/or manganese, all of which have been linked to bone health. So make sure that you continue to take your multi in addition to your calcium supplement—or pop a calcium supplement that provides vitamin D, magnesium, and zinc.

How do I know which supplement to take? When in doubt, choose a supplement made from calcium carbonate. It will deliver the most calcium per tablet,

Bone Up on Calcium-Rich Foods

It's not always convenient to meet your daily calcium requirements through food, but if you want to give it a try, here are the best food sources of calcium.

Food	Serving Size	Calcium (mg.)
Calcium-fortified orange juice	1 cup	440
Nonfat yogurt	1 cup	400
Calcium-fortified Lactaid milk, nonfat	1 cup	300
Milk, skim or 1 percent	1 cup	300
Low-fat Swiss cheese	1 slice	270
Bean curd (tofu) with calcium sulfate*	½ cup	260
Low-fat Cheddar cheese	1 slice	205
Salmon (canned, with edible bones)	3 oz.	205
Sardines (canned, with edible bones)	2 oz.	180
Collard greens (cooked)	½ cup	179
Roasted soy nuts*	½ cup	119
Frozen yogurt	½ cup	105
Dried beans (cooked)	1 cup	90
Kale (cooked)	½ cup	90
Butternut squash (cooked)	1 cup	84
Tempeh	½ cup	75
Broccoli (cooked)	½ cup	45

*Preliminary research indicates that besides being high in calcium, soy products contain plant chemicals—called isoflavones—that may help fight osteoporosis.

so you'll have fewer pills to swallow, and you'll end up paying less in the long run. In case you're wondering how the other options stack up, the table "How Much Calcium Is in That Supplement?" shows the most common types of calcium supplements, along with what percentage of each is actually calcium.

How do I know how much calcium a supplement contains? Sometimes it's tough to tell—even when you read the fine print on the side of the bottle. Take these two steps, however, and you should be able to ace any label.

1. Identify the milligrams of usable calcium. Ideally, but not often, the label will specify how much "elemental" (or usable) calcium the supplement contains. If it does, great. Skip to step 2. If it doesn't, simply look for the milligrams of plain "calcium" the supplement contains. Just be sure not to mistake plain calcium for calcium carbonate, calcium citrate, or other forms of calcium. If you do, you might think a supplement has more usable calcium than it actually does.

2. Determine how many tablets, capsules, wafers, or teaspoons you need to take to get the amount of usable calcium listed on the label. Don't assume you need only one tablet for this amount—we've seen as many as six required.

Can I get too much calcium? You sure can—and routinely overdosing on the mineral could make it difficult for your body to eliminate the calcium it doesn't need. So, although a regular calcium intake of 2,000 milligrams per day is safe, there's no reason to supplement with more than 1,500 milligrams unless your doctor prescribes it.

Which form of calcium will I absorb best? Truth is, brand doesn't matter (there's little difference in your body's ability to absorb different sources of calcium), but timing and dosage do. To maximize your absorption, take no more than 500 milligrams of calcium at a time and always take it with food.

What's the best time for me to take a calcium supplement? Anytime you can remember to pop a supplement is a great time. But just before you hit the hay may be best, if only to help keep your blood levels of calcium high during the night, when you're inactive and lose the most calcium.

Are there any foods or drugs that don't "mix" with calcium supplements? The only food that impairs calcium absorption enough to mention is wheat bran. Avoid taking a supplement with ultrahigh wheat bran cereals. On the flip side, calcium supplements can impair the absorption of other substances—namely iron and zinc in a multivitamin. So take your calcium supplements, multis, and certain drugs such as the antibiotic tetracycline separately, and be sure to tell your pharmacist that you're taking calcium when you have a prescription filled.

Will I hurt my stomach if I take calcium in the form of antacid calcium carbonate chewable tablets if I have no need for an antacid? Not a bit. Calcium carbonate chewables are no different from any other form of calcium carbonate supplements.

How Much Calcium Is in That Supplement?

Supplement	Percent Calcium
Calcium carbonate	40
Dicalcium phosphate	38
Bonemeal	31
Oyster shell	28
Dolomite	22
Calcium citrate	21
Calcium lactate	13
Calcium gluconate	9

The Latest on Drug Therapy

Estrogen replacement therapy (ERT) has been used successfully to help treat and prevent osteoporosis for decades. But in the past year, two terrific new drugs have become available. So now women—with the help of their doctors—can choose the medication best suited for their individual needs. "It's wonderful that we now have enough good drugs that we can think in terms of 'what's the best choice for you,'" says Dr. Siris. Here are the pros and cons of the drugs available.

Raloxifene (Evista). Approved by the U.S. Food and Drug Administration for *prevention* of osteoporosis (not as a treatment). This "designer estrogen" prevents bone loss quite well, though it's not as potent as conventional estrogen, says Dr. Siris. But it will be an attractive alternative to ERT and Fosamax.

Pros: Evista doesn't increase the risk of breast and uterine cancer, as ERT can. In fact, the drug may even help protect against breast cancer. And, unlike estrogen, it doesn't bring back a woman's period or cause breast tenderness.

Cons: Studies have proven that ERT reduces the risk of bone fracture and of heart attack. Although preliminary studies suggest Evista will have the same benefits, experts haven't yet done the long-term studies necessary to prove it. So a woman at high risk of heart disease might want to choose estrogen. What's more, Evista will not ease hot flashes and may even worsen them.

Estrogen Replacement Therapy. The best studied drug for the prevention and treatment of osteoporosis.

Pros: ERT increases bone mass even more than Evista. And it definitely lowers the risk of bone fracture and heart attack. Estrogen can ease menopausal hot flashes and vaginal dryness, and a small dose may offer bone protection: A two-year study reported in the *Archives of Internal Medicine* suggests that even half the normal dose of estrogen may halt bone thinning.

Cons: Long-term estrogen use seems to increase a woman's risk of breast cancer. And, when taken without progesterone, it can increase uterine cancer risk. It can also bring on menstruation and breast tenderness.

Alendronate (Fosamax). Approved for osteoporosis prevention and treatment in 1997.

Pros: Fosamax preserves bone mass as well as estrogen does and also reduces fracture risk. And it doesn't increase a woman's chances of developing breast cancer, as ERT can. According to Dr. Siris, if a woman is at high risk of osteoporosis, she might prefer Fosamax because, unlike Evista, it has been proven to lower fracture risk. Also, Fosamax, like estrogen, is an established treatment for osteoporosis.

Cons: The drug doesn't protect against heart disease or ease hot flashes. In addition, women with kidney disease, ulcers, or serious stomach or esophageal disorders can't take this drug.

New Options for Allergy Relief

O h, the coughing, the sneezing, the itchy, watery eyes. Is there no end in sight for people with allergies? Now there may be. Read on to discover some new options for relief.

Red Light Stops Sneezes Cold

No wonder Rudolph never sneezes. According to research done in Israel, red light directed into the nostrils can bring relief from allergy symptoms, reducing your trips to the doctor and the pharmacy. A study of this approach in 50 people with allergies found that 72 percent of them felt considerably better after red-laser phototherapy.

According to study author Ittai Neuman, M.D., the deck-of-cards-size device that produces the light should be available soon. The treatment uses a milder version of the red-light lasers used in surgery, and it's said to interfere with the body's release of histamines, the chemicals that cause allergic reactions.

"The research seems sound," says John Santilli, M.D., co-director of the Allergy Research Center at Bridgeport Hospital in Connecticut. "But there hasn't been any study yet of the long-term side effects," he cautions. "For now, our current allergy treatments are still the best and safest way to go."

Pet Owners Prefer to Live with Allergies

An allergy-free home appears to be no match for the cozy companionship of a dog or cat. Forced to choose between a teary goodbye and a lifetime of watery eyes, most allergic pet owners would opt for the latter, one study suggests.

For the study, Stanley Coren, Ph.D., a psychologist at the University of British Columbia in Vancouver, examined the case histories of 341 cat and dog owners with allergies to their pets. All had been advised by doctors to move their animal friends outside or bid them farewell altogether. A mere 21 percent complied. In a subgroup of 122 allergy patients who lost their pets from natural causes, 70 percent adopted another animal during the course of the study, despite the advice of their physicians. Companionship, Dr. Coren concluded, far outweighs physical discomfort for a vast majority of pet owners.

Pet allergies are brought on by proteins in animal saliva that are carried by shed fur and dander and inhaled by people. Cats are more likely than other species to trigger allergic reactions. The Asthma and Allergy Foundation of America estimates that 6 to 10 million Americans are allergic to cats. But even mice, hamsters, birds, and cockroaches can cause their share of sneezes.

If finding a new home for your pet is not an option for you, then you can take other steps to avoid allergic reactions. For example, make your bedroom off-limits to your pet; minimize or eliminate upholstered furniture and carpeting, which are havens for allergens; and outfit your vacuum with a microfiltration bag.

HEALTH FLASH

Antihistamine Spray Goes Right to the Source

Seasonal snifflers can now treat their noses without getting their whole bodies involved. The newest prescription antihistamine for allergic rhinitis (hay fever) has recently been released in the form of a spray. Azelastine HCl (Astelin) is the first and currently only antihistamine nasal spray that treats runny, sniffling, sneezing, and itchy noses directly at their source.

"Currently, all other antihistamines must be taken orally, which means that they are first absorbed into the bloodstream and then work systemically in the body," says Eli O. Meltzer, M.D., an allergy specialist at the University of California, San Diego. These include familiar over-the-counter (OTC) products, like Benadryl and Chlor-Trimeton, and newer prescription medicines, like Claritin and Allegra.

"Azelastine offers three potential benefits," says Dr. Meltzer. First, since it's administered as a nasal spray, you absorb less medication than you would when you swallow a pill. Second, you probably have a slightly faster onset of action. Third, it appears to cause less drowsiness than the older OTC products.

On the downside, one in five people complains of a bitter taste following its use. The aftertaste may be a deciding factor if you're already happy with your current antihistamine.

Azelastine can be used preventively, as needed, or continually. Unlike some prescription antihistamines, it does not have any known drug interactions that restrict its use.

A Recipe for Dust Mite Destruction

You can't see them, but you've heard of them: dust mites, those microscopic pests whose droppings make life miserable for people with asthma or allergies. Washing and drying clothing or bedding at hot temperatures effectively wipes out the allergens that mites leave, but the mites themselves live on to reproduce.

Now researchers in Australia have come up with a new technique: adding eucalyptus oil to your laundry. In a test, their approach slashed the population of mites in a wool blanket by 95 percent. Eucalyptus oil is generally available from stores that sell essential oils and natural products. Here's the mite-busting formula.

1. Mix one part detergent in three to five parts oil. If the detergent doesn't dissolve, you need to try another product.
2. Add a teaspoon of the mixture to an eight-ounce glass of water. The resulting milky solution should remain opaque for at least 10 minutes.
3. Once you have a "recipe" that passes steps one and two, put the mixture in a washer that has filled with water. (Never put the mixture in the washer without water. It could damage the drum.) Add your laundry and let it soak 30 to 60 minutes. Then continue with the wash cycle, as you normally do.

A once-a-year eucalyptus wash could be a bonus to the standard anti-mite tactics of cleaning bed linens weekly and keeping mattresses, pillows, and blankets encased.

10

Take Colds and Flu Off Your Calendar

With cold viruses lurking on everything from doorknobs to dollar bills, avoiding a cold can seem like dodging snowflakes in a blizzard. But the chances of keeping your nose clear during the winter months might actually not be so small. Here are ways that scientists have found to stop your next cold or at least soften its blow.

Invest in echinacea. Strange as it may sound, a purple member of the daisy family may head off your next cold. Thirty-two clinical trials indicate that the herb echinacea boosts the immune system. "It activates the specialized white blood cells that help destroy invading organisms such as cold viruses," says Varro E. Tyler, Ph.D., Sc.D., professor emeritus of pharmacognosy (the study of medicinal plants) at Purdue University in West Lafayette, Indiana. "It also inhibits an enzyme that causes the invading cold virus to pass from cell to cell."

Echinacea appears most effective when taken at the first signs of a cold. No harm has been associated with more extended use, but no benefits have been observed either. Dr. Tyler recommends buying the tablets or capsules (available in most health food stores) and following the dosage directions carefully. Check the label to make sure that the preparation you buy comes from either *Echinacea angustifolia* or *Echinacea purpurea* and that the mixture has been standardized.

Exercise, don't agonize. Forget "no pain, no gain." Moderate, not strenuous, exercise is the hero when it comes to cold-stopping powers. "Every time

Does Vitamin E Give Colds a Chill?

Want an immune system so big and bad that invading viruses "make its day"? A recent study suggests calling in the E squad—as in vitamin E supplements. In people 65 and over, those who took 200 international units (IU) of synthetic vitamin E daily for eight months had immune systems that were up to six times better prepared to battle nasty microbes compared with those in people who didn't take the vitamin. Vitamin E–takers also reported 30 percent fewer bouts with ills like colds, flu, and pneumonia, says vitamin E expert Simin Nikbin Meydani, Ph.D., of Tufts University in Medford, Massachusetts.

Will vitamin E benefit younger immune systems? That's still to be studied. But Dr. Meydani believes the results for people 65 and over are very encouraging, especially since there haven't been any harmful side effects.

Note: A group taking 800 IU of vitamin E got less immune upswing than the group taking 200 IU. Based on previous studies suggesting extra E may reduce risk of heart attack, consider taking 100 to 400 IU of vitamin E a day. If you are considering taking amounts above 200 IU, discuss this with your doctor first. One study using low-dose vitamin E supplements showed an increased risk of hemorrhagic stroke. You should also consult your doctor if you take aspirin or other blood-thinning medicine.

Can you get 200 IU of vitamin E in a good diet? In a word, no. Even if you used the richest sources of vitamin E, you'd need to eat huge quantities to reach 200 IU, such as six cups of wheat germ or nearly three cups of corn oil or a whopping five cups of peanut butter—which only has 725 grams of fat and a measly 8,000 calories!

HEALTH FLASH

you take a brisk walk, it increases the circulation of immune cells through your body," says David C. Nieman, D.H.Sc., professor of health and exercise science at Appalachian State University in Boone, North Carolina. That increase jacks up the chances that immune cells will meet up with and combat the cold virus. In three different studies, Dr. Nieman and his team of researchers found that women who walked fast enough to moderately boost their heart rates (30 to 45 minutes, five days a week) were sick half as often as women who remained sedentary.

But more is not better. If you exercise intensely for more than an hour, stress hormones kick in. "Those can suppress the immune system," says Dr. Nieman. "After a marathon, for example, a runner's risk of illness is six times greater than normal."

And don't think that one walk a month can bestow these protective powers. "A brisk walk gives a nice little boost to the immune system," says Dr. Nieman, "but only with near-daily activity."

Take zinc. It might sound unsavory, but taken in lozenge form, zinc appears to have some pretty impressive powers against colds. In a study at the Cleveland Clinic, 50 people with colds who sucked on lozenges every two hours that were packed with 13.3 milligrams of zinc kissed their symptoms goodbye in almost half the time of their placebo-popping counterparts.

Still, the study's author, Michael Macknin, M.D., is reluctant to say that his research is definitive. "It's exciting information, but until any medical treatment has been studied many times, you can't be confident that it definitely works," he says. In seven other studies, three reported similar benefits and four did not. Dr. Macknin suspects that different formulations may have affected the outcomes.

How zinc works is also uncertain, says Dr. Macknin, but he offers several theories. One is that zinc prevents the cold virus from hooking onto the respiratory tract and causing an infection. Another theory is that zinc may block the growth of the virus's outer coat, stunting its ability to multiply. Or zinc may stimulate production of the body's virus-fighting natural substance, interferon, or it may shore up cell membranes, making them less vulnerable to viral infection in the first place.

Zinc lozenges (the most common brand name is Cold-Eeze) are available in most drug, grocery, and health food stores. Zinc lozenges have some side effects: About 80 percent of the people who tried them said that the lozenges had an unpleasant aftertaste, and 20 percent were nauseated. To combat nausea, Dr. Macknin recommends sucking the lozenges on a full stomach.

Caution: Only use zinc lozenges when you have a cold, not on a regular basis. Too much zinc can actually impair immune system functioning.

Make a habit of hand washing. Washing your hands as often as possible is the first line of defense against colds, says cold expert George L. Kirkpatrick, M.D., clinical associate professor of emergency medicine at the University of South Alabama in Mobile. But we're not talking about just any kind of hand washing. According to a 1997 study by a researcher at Purdue University Calumet in Hammond, Indiana, the proper hand-washing technique is equally important. (No quick rinses allowed here.) A group of teachers and school-age children who were taught to wash their hands thoroughly and properly ended up getting fewer colds during a 10-week peak-cold-season period than did a similar group who washed their hands in the usual hurried manner.

"Washing properly means wetting your hands with water and lathering up with an antibacterial soap," says Dr. Kirkpatrick. "Rub all the surfaces of both hands together, including the insides of your fingers, for at least two minutes. Then go up your wrist, and then pick under your fingernails to clean out the debris." Dr. Kirkpatrick washes his hands approximately every five minutes when doing patient care in the emergency room, but unless you're a doctor, every five minutes probably doesn't fit your schedule. Aim for a scrub before and after hand contact and especially before and after you eat and after changing baby diapers or going to the bathroom. And teach all family members to wash their hands after they sneeze or cough into them.

Keep your distance. It's a maxim most of us learned at Mom's knee, but it seems that Mom (again) was right: The basic way to avoid a cold is to avoid people with colds. Each time a cold victim sneezes or speaks, she sends volleys of viral water droplets through the air, as far as 30 feet. Even a well-intended handshake can pass along a cold virus. "If your immune system is strong, you may not get a cold," says Dr. Kirkpatrick. "But you're now carrying the virus. Touch your child, she gets a cold, and then you wonder where she got it."

The most critical period to avoid contact, according to Jack M. Gwaltney Jr., M.D., head of the division of epidemiology and virology at the University of Virginia Health Sciences Center in Charlottesville and a leader in cold research for more than 30 years, is the first two to three days that the person has symptoms. The best ploy is to be a little paranoid: If a co-worker starts sniffling or sounds a bit hoarse, keep your distance for a couple of days.

Unfortunately, despite what you may have heard, the no-contact edict even applies to your significant other. While saliva has special properties that can inhibit the spread of cold viruses, you don't want to kiss someone who is in the throes of a cold. "It's common sense to wait a few days to avoid coming in contact with the virus," says Thomas Petro, Ph.D., associate professor of microbiology at the University of Nebraska College of Dentistry in Lincoln.

So do you avoid all contact with other people? Of course not. We need to be with people. In fact, at least one recent study suggests that having a wide variety of friends can help reduce the number of colds we get. Still, we can reduce our chances of sharing their germs or spreading ours. Teach your children to cover their mouths and noses with tissues every time they cough or sneeze, and to toss the tissues and wash their hands afterward. Make sure the adults in the family follow this routine as well. In addition, "it's probably worthwhile to wipe off countertops and tables with disinfectant immediately before everyone congregates for meals since the germs will repopulate the surfaces in about 30 minutes," says Dr. Kirkpatrick. "And don't share toothbrushes, drinking glasses, or teacups." Other smarts: Shop when crowds are smallest. And postpone your child's play date until Billy is over his cold.

Enjoy the great outdoors. Get caught in the cold and you'll catch a cold—how many times have we heard that one? Guess what? According to Dr. Gwaltney, there's no evidence that cooling the body induces a cold or that cold viruses thrive in cold weather. On the contrary, the reason we suffer more colds in the winter months is that we spend more time indoors, in enclosed quarters and in close contact with others. Go outside and you may actually reduce your risk of becoming infected.

Beware of air travel. One of the easiest places to pick up a cold is in an airplane cabin. The stagnant air is known for carrying viruses. If you have to fly, drink plenty of fluids.

Sleep eight hours a night. Researchers have not directly proven that sleep deprivation causes more colds, but Michael Irwin, M.D., professor of psychiatry at the University of California, San Diego, School of Medicine, has found that even a modest disturbance of sleep alters the body's immune function. "Sleep loss of three to four hours can cause a 50 percent decline in immune response," he says.

Good, but Not Guaranteed

Here are some cold-busters you may be familiar with. While they work for some people, there's no guarantee they will keep you safe from lurking cold viruses.

Take vitamin C. Once you have a cold, vitamin C can help reduce the duration and severity of your symptoms. That's what one Finnish researcher found when he analyzed and compared the results of numerous vitamin C studies. "Researchers are just beginning to understand how it affects our immune systems," says Barbara Levine, R.D., Ph.D., associate clinical professor of nutrition in medicine at Cornell University Medical College in New York City. "Many of the studies that have been done have not been well-controlled or well-done." Plus, when it comes to actually preventing colds, vitamin C may fall short for most of us. Some Finnish research suggests that vitamin C's cold-stopping power is limited to just a few groups of people, such as strenuous exercisers or people whose vitamin C intake is already low. But if you want to increase your vitamin C intake, make sure that you eat plenty of fresh fruits and vegetables. Good sources of C include oranges, strawberries, kiwifruit, broccoli, tomatoes, and peppers.

Make more friends. The more varied and abundant your social ties, the safer you may be from a cold, suggests a study done by Carnegie Mellon University in Pittsburgh. Of 276 adults exposed to cold viruses, those with the widest variety of social contacts also had the lowest cold risk—half that of their counterparts who were the least social. It may be that a broad spectrum of friends (provided they cover their sneezes) may help us deal more effectively with stresses that lower immunity.

Gargle twice a day. A study from Japan found that workers who gargled three times daily over a three-month period reported fewer colds, took less medication, and were less likely to call in sick than those who didn't gargle. You probably shouldn't gargle more than that, however. The preventive value of gargling is temporary, and too much can actually kill good microbes in your mouth, explains Dr. Petro.

To maintain the proper pH in your mouth, Dr. Petro advises gargling twice a day with a mouthwash that has antimicrobial properties. Look for ones with the word *antiseptic* on the label.

Do things that make you happy. The relationship between daily events and the immune system has been studied by Arthur A. Stone, Ph.D., a psychologist at the State University of New York at Stony Brook. He found that desirable daily events that boost your mood (such as quality time with your kids, a good meeting with your boss, or an hour with a good book) have a positive effect on the immune system, while undesirable events that deflate your mood (such as a fight with your mate, a flat tire, or a really bad hair day) have a negative impact.

"We found that undesirable events peaked and desirable events hit a trough about 3½ days before the onset of a cold," says Dr. Stone. The best advice to avoid getting sick: Reduce the number of undesirable events in your life as much as you can, and try not to let those that do happen bug you so much.

11

Help for an Aching Head

We all know the sensation: a dull throbbing at the back of your head, just above your neck. Or the sense that someone is tightening a belt around your forehead and temples. Or maybe it's an excruciating pain above one eye—then both.

Chronic headaches plague 45 million Americans. As a nation, we're likely to spend a staggering $4 billion on over-the-counter pain relievers this year and lose 157 million workdays to the everyday headache.

Increasingly, however, headache sufferers are taking charge of their pain. When aspirin and ibuprofen fail, the solution isn't necessarily a day home in bed in a darkened room. For people who get migraines, new prescription drugs, such as Imitrex, have been very effective at stopping a headache in its early stages, while Depakote seems to be a potent preventive. Unfortunately, these pills can be costly and, as with any powerful drug, there can be side effects: nausea, muscle spasms in the neck, and "rebound" headaches.

Consequently, some headache sufferers are turning to alternative, all-natural avenues for relief. Sometimes the remedy is as simple as a little lavender oil on the temples or a warm mug of ginger tea; sometimes it's more complex, such as chiropractics with a "neuroemotional component," for example, or a weekly session with a trained acupuncturist.

Of course, none of these "cures" works for everybody; it's also important to note that the National Headache Foundation (NHF) is wary of all alternative-healing approaches—with the notable exception of biofeedback. "You're going to find anecdotal incidents where aromatherapy or homeopathy or herbal medicine work, but they're not consistent," says Seymour Diamond, M.D., chairman of the NHF. "I'm not opposed to anything that works," he says, "but don't expect miracles from most [alternative] treatments."

So before you start steeping your ginger tea, a quick primer on headaches is in order.

Identify Your Headache

Marc Sharfman, M.D., a headache specialist at Winter Park Memorial Hospital in Winter Park, Florida, treats headaches with both conventional drugs and a somewhat less conventional regimen of massage, physical therapy, nutritional therapy, and biofeedback. Once he has established that there is no identifiable cause—such as a sinus infection, an aneurysm, or a brain tumor—he classifies the headache as one of three types: tension, migraine, or cluster.

Tension headaches. Most of us have experienced these headaches, which are usually triggered by stress. The stress causes the muscles in the neck, scalp, or face to contract, which in turn results in a headache.

Migraine headaches. According to the NHF, 17 million of us know too well what a migraine feels like: pulsating pain, nausea, a tremendous sensitivity to light and noise—often preceded by a flashing light or "aura." Migraines are also called vascular headaches because the blood vessels have become dilated and inflamed. The cause? Current theory holds that the body is releasing too much or too little of certain natural anti-inflammatories, like serotonin. Some migraines are also hereditary and have been mapped to a specific chromosome.

Cluster headaches. These headaches, which, fortunately, few of us have to endure, come in groups. Several times a day for weeks, or even months, these vascular headaches will descend like locusts, usually afflicting one side of the head. Then, just as suddenly as they began, they stop. Sometimes they're gone for months, sometimes forever. Their onset may be linked to the body's level of serotonin, but it may also be caused by a sudden alteration in a person's circadian rhythms (switching from a day shift to a night shift, for example).

Most headaches are not caused by a tumor or disease, Dr. Sharfman says, but he recommends strongly that you "rule out these organic causes before beginning any sort of nonmedical approach." In other words, consult a doctor before pursuing any of these treatments.

That caveat noted, here are several alternative ways to combat headache pain. A few of them have great support in the traditional medical community, while others elicit rolled eyes and raised eyebrows from conventional M.D.'s. All, however, are safe and free from side effects. Even if they don't heal that headache, they probably won't make it worse.

Heal Yourself with Biofeedback

Biofeedback teaches a person to control functions of her autonomic (or involuntary) nervous system such as skin temperature, blood pressure, and heartbeat. With the help of instruments that monitor skin temperature, blood pressure, or muscle tension, people literally train themselves to raise or lower their body temperatures or relax their muscles. The techniques include relaxation and breathing exercises and the development of guided images focusing on warmth and relaxation.

Clinical studies have demonstrated consistently that people can relax their muscles or change their body temperatures enough to stop a headache in its tracks. (Skin temperature is an indicator of how dilated the veins are in our bodies, and many headaches are the result of the blood vessels becoming overly dilated.)

Biofeedback is at once so successful and so noninvasive that it's actually Dr. Sharfman's treatment of choice for pregnant women at the Headache and Neurological Treatment Institute, also in Winter Park. But biofeedback takes time to learn, and then requires continual practice. At the very least, a person must do biofeedback exercises two or three times every day.

Florida photographer Kathleen Overchuck, 25, one of Dr. Sharfman's patients, doesn't mind. Granted, she has covered the walls of her home with one-inch green dots as a reminder to do her exercises, which involve relaxing her forehead and jaw. But that, in her mind, is a small price to pay for the dramatic decrease in both the frequency and the severity of her headaches. She used to face at least three migraines a week, and now it's rarely more than one.

Many mainstream physicians and neurologists offer biofeedback training. To learn more about it, contact the National Headache Foundation. You can obtain the organization's 800 number by calling toll-free directory assistance.

Get Needled

We all have a vision in our minds when we see the word *acupuncture:* a human porcupine, or a prone body pierced with more needles than a pin cushion. But it's considerably more refined than that, says Los Angeles acupuncturist and Oriental medicine doctor Jocelyne Eberstein. Thin needles are inserted along specific energy pathways that Oriental medicine doctors believe course throughout the body. This stimulates the circulation of energy and releases the body's painkilling endorphins. Acupuncture is, in the opinion of most practitioners, excellent at relieving tension and stress—the source, after all, of a great many headaches.

At her holistic clinic, Eberstein frequently treats her headache patients with acupuncture because "it often gives the first immediate relief." With regular treatment, however, she says it can eliminate headaches long-term. Patients should anticipate a month of treatment for every year they've been in pain, with one or more acupuncture sessions a week. But, she adds, "even if it's been a lifetime of pain, a person will usually start feeling some relief within three to six months."

To learn more about this 3,000-year-old technique, contact the American Association of Oriental Medicine at 433 Front Street, Catasauqua, PA 18032, or the National Acupuncture and Oriental Medicine Alliance at 14637 Starr Road SE, Olalla, WA 98359.

Try "Tennis Ball" Acupressure

Barbara Kreiling, a certified massage therapist in a suburb of Chicago, treats many of her clients who have tension headaches and migraines with acupressure—acupuncture, essentially, without the needles. At the very same points on the skin where an acupuncturist will insert needles to relieve pain, Kreiling applies gentle finger pressure.

Many of her clients are busy executives who struggle constantly with tension headaches, especially when they're on the road and far from Kreiling's powerful fingers and hands. Her solution for them?

"I have them take two soft tennis balls with them when they travel," she says. "When they're in their hotel rooms, they lie on their backs on a carpeted part of the floor and place the tennis balls side by side under the back of their heads—just below the base of the skull, where the bone starts to curl in. And then they relax. The weight of the head against the tennis balls does all the work. Five minutes is often enough to make the headache go away."

This technique works best as an adjunct to regular acupressure massage, but it can help anyone coping with a tension headache, according to Kreiling. To find a certified therapist near you, contact the Jin Shin Do Foundation for Bodymind Acupressure at P. O. Box 1097, Felten, CA 95018.

Change Your Diet

Lorilee Schoenbeck, a naturopathic physician in Shelburne, Vermont, advises migraine sufferers to avoid foods that have been shown to trigger that kind of headache: alcohol (especially red wine), cheese, and caffeine (even from chocolate). A small study at Loma Linda University also suggests that reducing fat intake decreases both the frequency and the pain of headaches for people who get migraines.

Food allergies are also often a cause of chronic headache pain. Unfortunately, determining if you're allergic to a specific food—dairy products, perhaps, or the gluten found in such grains as wheat, barley, and rye—is more complex than simply tracking whether a headache starts after you finish that Swiss cheese on rye. Often the allergens won't have an effect until they've been in your blood for one to four days. If you suspect a food allergy is at the root of your problems, Schoenbeck recommends visiting your physician for a food allergy blood test or skin-prick test.

Get Rolfed

Rolfing, a form of massage that involves manipulation of the connective tissue within the body to "reshape" the body's architecture, has gotten a bad rap in the last decade, according to Rolfer Kristen Kuester of Santa Fe, New Mexico. "It has this reputation for being painful," she says, "but it has changed so much in the last 15 years. I don't think my work hurts."

Client Loretta Lopez, 30, agrees. She began seeing Kuester after an automobile accident had left her with migrainelike headaches that would lodge just above her eyes at night and keep her from sleeping. After a few sessions, her headaches were gone. In addition to the actual Rolfing massages, Kuester also offered her important tips on how to walk, stand, and sit properly, which Lopez thinks have also helped keep her headache-free. Other postural therapies, like the Alexander Technique, have also proved successful in giving relief to people with chronic headaches.

To learn more about Rolfing or to find a certified Rolfer near you, contact the Rolf Institute at 205 Canyon Boulevard, Boulder, CO 80302.

Get Your Spine and Mind Working As One

For the first time in her adult life, 57-year-old Bonnie Cantrell is finding relief from the headaches that were not just painful but disabling. The result of being kicked in the head by a horse after the animal threw her, Cantrell's headaches were so agonizing that she eventually gave up the job she loved in public affairs with the NASA Jet Propulsion Laboratory to lie in her bedroom in the dark.

Her panacea arrived in the hands of Burbank, California, chiropractor Muffit Jensen—who didn't simply "crack" bones or "manipulate" the spine; she offered Cantrell chiropractic treatment with a "neuroemotional component." In addition to giving her deep muscle massages and attempting to realign the vertebrae in her back, the chiropractor also had Cantrell "reenact" her fall from the horse. While Cantrell, wearing her riding boots, jeans, and a cowboy shirt, lay in hay on the floor in her chiropractor's office, the chiropractor rocked Cantrell's head in her hands, trying to help the woman's body "release" the pain and terror of the riding disaster.

Cantrell's headaches have since plummeted from five or six every day to only one or two a week, and that single headache is considerably less debilitating.

Dr. Jensen explains that she is merely one of a growing number of chiropractors who approach the body from an emotional and biochemical perspective as well as a structural one. "Sometimes we still address a headache structurally—a thrust here, a tender touch there," she says. "But the best way to deal with a headache is to find its root cause: a fall, an emotional trauma. They can all contribute to vertebral misalignment—and pain."

To find a chiropractor near you, write to the American Chiropractic Association at 1701 Clarendon Boulevard, Arlington, VA 22209. Then ask the practitioner if she is a neuroemotional chiropractor.

Steep a Cup of Ginger Tea

Although acupuncturist and Oriental medicine doctor Eberstein believes that it's important to understand what's triggering a headache and try to eliminate those root causes, she has also found that ginger tea helps reduce headache pain.

Her recipe: "Grate a teaspoon of fresh ginger into a cup, and pour boiling water on it. Let it steep for five minutes. When you sip it, the ginger moves the chi—or vital force—in our bodies," she says. Getting the chi moving is crucial because pain such as tension headaches is caused by a chi blockage, she explains. "That knot in your shoulders? That's a chi blockage."

Savor the Smell of Essential Oil

Aromatherapy, or the use of the essential oils from plants, has done for upstate New York retired school nurse and teacher Mary Jane Stanley, 42, what conventional painkillers could not. It has relieved the periodic headaches she's endured since she was diagnosed with a golf ball–size brain tumor in 1991. Though the tumor was benign, surgeons were only able to remove 90 percent of the mass, and the part that remained—along with nerve damage caused during surgery—continued to cause her often profound discomfort.

Not any more. Now Stanley uses a special blend of oils prepared by Burlington, Vermont, aromatherapist Wendy Dorsey. She also uses the headache "staples" in an aromatherapist's arsenal: a little peppermint on the back of the neck when she feels a headache commencing or a drop of lavender on the temples. Occasionally, Stanley adds a few drops of chamomile to her bath or fills her home with aromas via a diffuser that warms the oil.

Aromatherapy can be extremely potent, says Dorsey, because "our sense of smell is one of our primary survival mechanisms. The plants that aromatherapists use have hundreds of chemical constituents that work in a variety of ways in our bodies."

Grapefruit, for example, seems to signal the release of serotonin into the bloodstream, while chamomile acts as an anti-inflammatory. And peppermint, an aromatherapist's anti-headache mainstay, has a chemical in it called terpene, which seems to have an analgesic effect when dabbed on the skin.

Is Your Painkiller Making Your Head Hurt?

Over-the-counter (OTC) pills that you take to get rid of headaches can actually make headaches worse if you take them too often, according to Harvard neurologist Nathaniel Katz, M.D.

"At least 2 to 3 percent of the population in this country—millions of people—may use large quantities of pain medications for headache control," says Ninan T. Mathew, M.D., director of the Houston Headache Clinic. Painkillers containing caffeine are prime causes of rebound headache because caffeine withdrawal itself triggers headache.

How do you know whether the headaches you have are caused by the very painkillers you're taking to relieve them? Look for these warning signs.

❖ You're taking painkillers for migraine or tension headaches more than two or three days a week on a regular basis. This is the limit most headache experts set for safety of either prescription or OTC headache medicines. "If you take analgesics more than a couple of times a week for migraine or related headaches, you're vulnerable to having the headache escalate in frequency and become more difficult to treat," says rebound headache expert Joel R. Saper, M.D., director of the Michigan Head Pain and Neurological Institute in Ann Arbor.

❖ You can't leave the house without a bottle of painkillers in your purse or briefcase.

❖ You're buying aspirin or acetaminophen as often as you buy *TV Guide* or *Newsweek*.

❖ When you sleep late on weekends, you wake up with a pounding headache—your body demanding its fix.

❖ You have a headache almost daily or get one at the slightest mentally or physically stressful situation.

❖ Pills don't get rid of the pain—but they take the edge off. "That phrase—'take the edge off'—should set off a lightbulb that what you're dealing with is withdrawal and rebound," says Glen Solomon, M.D., former head of the headache section at the Cleveland Clinic. "It's the universal rebound statement."

The only way for the pain machine in your brain to reset itself is to stop feeding it pills. Complete resetting can take anywhere from 4 to 12 weeks, says Fred Sheftell, M.D., co-director of the New England Center for Headache in Stamford, Connecticut, and co-author of *Headache Relief for Women*. That usually means about a week to 10 days of increased headaches.

"The important thing to remember is that if you can just manage to stay off daily pain medicine, you'll feel much better after two to three weeks," says Dr. Mathew.

12 More Drug-Free Ways to Heal Your Head

Before you go to the medicine chest for another battle with a childproof cap, here are 12 drug-free, effective ways to make that headache vanish.

1. Put your pain on ice. Good old frozen water. It's natural. It's free (for the most part). And if you put it on your head when you have a headache, it's one of the fastest ways to stop the hurting. At the first sign of pain, top your forehead with an ice pack or a bag of frozen vegetables wrapped in a towel.

2. Turn up the heat. If your headache is the result of tension, you may want to opt for heat treatment instead of ice. When you're tense, your neck muscles tighten and your arteries constrict, reducing the flow of blood to your brain and causing a tension headache. Heat helps to soothe muscles and increase blood supply. Try a heating pad at the back of your head, a long hot shower (aim the spray at the back of your neck), or a hot bath.

3. Wrap it up. "The old business of Grandmother tying a cloth tightly around her head has some merit to it," says Glen Solomon, M.D., former head of the headache section at the Cleveland Clinic. "It decreases the blood flow to the scalp and lessens the throbbing and pounding of a migraine," he explains. A headband wrapped around your forehead and the base of your skull has the same effect.

4. Rub it the right way. Massage your head with your fingertips as if you were washing your hair. If you have short hair, place a natural-bristle hairbrush at your temple above your eyebrows, and gradually move it toward the back of your head in slow circles.

5. Take matters into your own hands. "You can 'massage' away headaches by pushing on certain acupressure spots," says Fred Sheftell, M.D., co-director of the New England Center for Headache in Stamford, Connecticut, and co-author of *Headache Relief for Women*. "One way is to tightly squeeze the web of skin between your thumb and forefinger. Another area is the ridge between your neck and the back of your head (approximately parallel with your earlobes)." Also try massaging the top of your foot, the outside of your shin (below the knee), or your Achilles tendon.

To learn more about aromatherapy, contact the National Association for Holistic Aromatherapy at P.O. Box 17622, Boulder, CO 80308.

Try a Natural Pain Reliever

For an occasional headache, an over-the-counter drugstore pain reliever often does the trick. But if used frequently—just three or four times a week—

6. Take a deep breath. If you find that you're a little on edge, deep breathing can relieve your tension. "You're doing it right," Dr. Sheftell says, "if your stomach is moving more than your chest."

7. Seek some peace and quiet. "Probably the simplest thing you can do to feel better is to go to a dark, quiet room and lie down," says Dr. Solomon. "That's because any kind of movement can aggravate a headache, so anything you can do to keep your neck muscles from tightening will help." Why a dark, quiet room? Even small headaches make you more sensitive to light and noise.

8. Get a move on. If the headache isn't too severe, go for a walk. Aerobic exercise not only helps you relax but also boosts your levels of endorphin, brain chemicals that diminish pain.

9. Roll in the hay. Making love may be a tonic for head pain. Research done at Southern Illinois University School of Medicine shows that most women get full or partial headache relief from having sex.

10. Get some shut-eye. A lot of folks are able to sleep off a headache, says Ninan T. Mathew, M.D., director of the Houston Headache Clinic. Sleeping on your back is probably your best bet, because sleeping in an awkward position or on your stomach contracts your neck muscles, which may prolong your head pain.

11. Stand tall. Posture plays a key role in tension headaches. Avoid leaning or tilting your head to one side since these positions tighten your neck muscles.

12. Make faces. The secret is in the muscles' movement. Try the following exercises, courtesy of Harry C. Ehrmantrout, Ph.D., author of *Headaches: The Drugless Way to Lasting Relief*, to relieve the pain. Practice them now, then do them at the first sign of a headache: Raise your eyebrows, first both, then separately. Squint your eyes closed, first both, then each separately. Frown deeply. Yawn wide. Move your jaw from side to side. Wrinkle your nose. Then, make faces (you can ad-lib this one).

analgesic painkillers, such as aspirin and ibuprofen, may actually exacerbate both the frequency and discomfort of headaches. This "analgesic rebound" is a common ailment among headache sufferers.

One solution may be to take a pain reliever that's made from herbs or trees. Naturopath Schoenbeck has had success treating migraines with an extract that's made from the 200-million-year-old ginkgo tree. The ginkgo stabilizes the blood vessels in the brain after the body's release of its natural inflammatories has caused the vessels to swell. She also prescribes valerian root, a natural muscle relaxer, to help ease tension headaches.

Many people who get headaches swear by a pain reliever made from feverfew, a garden plant that's a part of the chrysanthemum family. The plant decreases the body's secretion of serotonin, which in turn decreases the likelihood that the blood vessels will dilate. Feverfew isn't a silver bullet once a headache has started, however; instead, it's a preventive that sufferers need to take every day, like a vitamin or supplement. Moreover, it takes time before it will start to have a beneficial effect: Patients often take feverfew for three months before they notice a change, in rare cases coping at first with the side effect of a queasy stomach.

Finally, there is one other role plants can play in pain relief. If your headaches are linked to your hormones, certain plants can help level your body's chemical roller coaster. To learn if your headaches are hormonal, record on a calendar for a few months exactly when your headaches are occurring, and note if they come at the same time every month—perhaps premenstrually, midcycle (at ovulation), or during menses.

For relief, naturopaths like Schoenbeck recommend the roots from burdock, dandelion, or yellowdock, because they aid in the body's metabolism of cholesterol, and hormones have a cholesterol base. The right dosage will help restore the delicate hormonal balance that has been toppled during the cycle. These plants are available in health food stores as pills and teas—as are most natural pain relievers. But before you experiment with them, consult with a conventional or naturopathic physician. It's not that any of these plants are dangerous, but figuring out how much to take is more complicated than simply reading the label.

Help Yourself to More Sleep

W e'd like you to try something. It's simple, painless—even free. Doing it will make you feel and function better. Want to give it a shot? Here goes: Go to your bedroom. Lie down. Close your eyes. Fall asleep.

We know that may sound ridiculous. After all, who gets enough sleep? Everybody you know has the same lifestyle—too many hours at work, way too many responsibilities at home. No one gets a full eight hours. And it's not a big deal.

Well, that might not be the case. Recent research suggests that a lack of sleep can interfere with the immune system, short-circuit the growth of muscle and bone, and raise your blood pressure. Yet Americans sleep 20 percent less than their ancestors did a century ago, and the National Commission on Sleep Disorders Research estimates that no fewer than 60 million of us are chronically sleep-deprived.

You know the saying, "If you snooze, you lose"? Well, we're not snoozing, but we're definitely losing. Lack of shut-eye might be the biggest health problem in America—and we're too tired to acknowledge it.

Eight Is Enough

Individual demands vary, of course, but research suggests that the average person needs to get at least 8 hours of shut-eye each night—and she needs it regularly. According to one report from the Dayton Veterans Administration Hospital in Ohio, reducing sleep by just 1½ hours for a single night can lower daytime alertness by up to 33 percent. And Michael Bonnet, Ph.D., director of the hospital's sleep laboratory, notes that 4 hours of sleep loss, or two days in a row of sleeping just 6 hours a night, can slow reaction times by 10 to 15 percent. But boost that sleep time to a full 8 hours, and here's what it can do for you.

Build and repair your body. During deep sleep, our bodies circulate 70 percent of our daily dose of human growth hormone, which is used to repair skin and build muscle and bone.

Improve your defenses. A study from the University of California, San Diego, showed that, after missing five hours of sleep, healthy volunteers produced fewer disease-fighting immune cells.

Lower your blood pressure. Some doctors still question these results, but a

Sheepless Sleep

It's the night before your first tennis match in ages. You hit the hay early, but at 3:00 A.M., you're still wide awake. What do you do? Simply curl up on your right side. "Your heart will fall away from your chest wall, not into it, as it beats," explains Arnie Barker, M.D., a San Diego–based family practitioner and champion cyclist.

"This simple shift can make all the difference if your pulse is pumped up with performance anxiety. Think about it—a pounding heart can keep anyone awake. Why give it something to pound against?"

small study out of Japan showed that people who slept just 3.6 hours a night had significantly higher blood pressure the next day.

Hone your brain. Our ability to do useful mental work declines by 25 percent every successive 24 hours we're awake, say scientists at the Walter Reed Army Institute of Research in Washington, D.C.

Lift your mood. A recent study conducted at Brigham and Women's Hospital in Boston showed that volunteers felt happier if they slept in sync with their bodies' internal clocks.

So why don't we all relax and sleep more? Conventional wisdom says that's what lazy people do when they're busy not working.

A Bad Reputation In Bed

"There's almost a sense of shame about sleep in this country," says Rubin Naiman, Ph.D., a clinical health psychologist and director of Somna Sleep Health Associates in Tucson, Arizona. "Think of how often you're awakened by a late-night or early-morning phone call, only to be asked, 'Were you sleeping?' The most common response is to deny it." Or you might explain that you were up late with a report or a sick child, so the caller will think you deserved the extra time in bed.

Odds are, you deserve much more. Consider, for a moment, your nightly routine. "It ought to take you at least 5 to 10 minutes to fall asleep," says Dr. Naiman. "But many folks say, 'I'm a good sleeper. My head hits the pillow, and I'm out.' That's like somebody saying, 'I'm a good eater. I sit down to my breakfast, and it's gone in 30 seconds.' Inhaling your food isn't a sign of a good eater. It's a sign of someone who's starving." Here are six other symptoms of the sleep-starved.

1. You wake with an alarm clock, but only after repeatedly pounding the snooze button.

Get Up Earlier on the Weekends

Have you ever wondered why your Monday morning "rise and shine" feels more like a "groan and droop"? If so, you're not alone. One-third of Americans suffer from excessive daytime sleepiness, according to a recent Gallup poll sponsored by the National Sleep Foundation. One culprit could be your weekend sleep habits: Staying up late and sleeping in on Saturday and Sunday can make it hard to get up early on Monday.

Yeah, we know luxuriating under the covers is sweet payback for being rudely buzzed awake for five mornings in a row. But your body has a natural wake-up time attuned to the ebb and flow of the hormone cortisol. Sleeping late on the weekend throws your cortisol rhythm out of whack.

"When you go to bed later on Friday and Saturday night and rise later on Saturday and Sunday morning, your body gets used to a different sleep cycle," explains Timothy Roehrs, Ph.D., director of research at the Sleep Disorders and Research Center at the Henry Ford Hospital in Detroit. "By Monday morning, your alarm clock may wake you as much as two hours earlier than your body is used to."

If you need your weekends to catch up on sleep, try bedding down earlier or taking a midday nap, Dr. Roehrs recommends. "Be sure not to nap within four hours of your normal bedtime," he cautions. "That can disrupt nighttime sleep."

2. You remember having more energy in your well-rested past.
3. Your memory and thinking aren't as sharp as they used to be.
4. You sleep late on weekends. Biologically, this makes as much sense as breathing more on the weekends.
5. You rely on coffee, tea, nicotine, or other stimulants to get you through the day.
6. You fall asleep when you're bored.

"Most everybody will tell you that boredom makes them sleepy," observes Thomas Roth, Ph.D., director of the sleep disorders and research department at Henry Ford Hospital in Detroit. "This simply means that they're sleep-deprived. Their bodies are seizing the moment, and that's not productive. A well-rested person who's bored is going to find something interesting and challenging to do."

Give It a Rest

"If we operated machinery the way we routinely operate the human body, we'd be accused of reckless endangerment," says James Maas, Ph.D., professor of psychology and sleep researcher at Cornell University in Ithaca, New York, and author of *The Sleep Advantage*. "As a society, we have to make sleep a priority."

Here's how to put sleep back on your A-list and improve your health and productivity.

Keep regular hours. Let your VCR catch the late-night shows and do your best to crawl into and out of bed at the same time every day. (Yes, that means Saturday and Sunday, too.)

Soak before you snooze. Try taking a warm 15-minute bath just before you hit the hay. After you step out of the water and cool off a bit, your body temperature will drop, which is a natural sleep-inducer.

Hit the gym. A workout makes you tired. Get it? And as long as you don't reach for the dumbbells too close to bedtime (leave at least three hours between counting reps and counting sheep), the exertion will improve the quality of your sleep.

Stay away from sleeping pills. They're addictive and won't induce the deep sleep you need.

Give yourself 30 minutes to fall asleep. If that's not enough, crawl out of bed and do something relaxing, then try again when you're feeling drowsy.

Although it may take a little while to settle into your natural sleep pattern, once you do, you have it made. In fact, most experts estimate that it takes just a few days of purposeful sleeping to recover from chronic deprivation. "Sleep debt is like that loan you took from your parents in college," says Dr. Naiman. "You make a few payments, then you're forgiven the rest."

13 Supercharge Your Energy Now

Why is it that some people can barely drag themselves through the workday while others seem to have zip to spare?

In a word: energy. "Energy is a measure of physical and emotional vigor that causes us both to want and be able to take on many activities—those that provoke thought and those that require physical strength," says Miriam Nelson, Ph.D., associate chief of the Human Physiology Laboratory at the Jean Mayer USDA Human Nutrition Research Center on Aging at Tufts University in Medford, Massachusetts.

Most everyone has a sense of what energy feels like, but where does it come from?

The short answer is sugar—specifically, its simplest form, glucose. As we all learned in school, the food we eat gets converted into glucose, which is the brain's primary energy source and the most common, efficient substance from which all of our body's cells obtain energy. A single molecule of glucose can trigger the production of up to 38 molecules of ATP, a chemical that scientists call the energy molecule since nearly all processes and reactions in the body—from breathing to digesting, winking to shooting baskets—are fueled by it. Without ATP, cells lock up and muscles stiffen, unable to carry out normal functions. (This accounts for the rigor mortis effect in a lifeless body, which no longer produces ATP.)

Generally speaking, our personal energy stores are largely determined by

Exhaustion Is Hazardous to Your Health

A good night's sleep is a must for optimum energy. Without adequate shut-eye, you feel exhausted and unable to function.

Scientists are just beginning to understand how significant this impairment can be. At least one study has suggested that lack of sleep can hinder performance just as much as consuming alcohol.

The two-part study, conducted at the University of Southern Australia, involved a group of 40 medical students. In the first part, the students had to stay awake for 28 hours straight. In the second part, they kept their regular sleep schedules, but upon waking, they drank a shot of grain alcohol every 30 minutes until their blood alcohol levels reached 0.10. (This is considered the legal limit for drunk driving in most states.) During each segment, researchers periodically evaluated the students' eye-hand coordination using a test that simulated basic driving skills.

After 19 hours without sleep, the students performed as though they had consumed a couple of drinks. After 24 hours, their eye-hand coordination was as poor as when they were legally drunk. The longer the students stayed awake, the more their performance deteriorated.

These findings have already proven pivotal in several court cases in Australia. Judges there are holding employers responsible for automobile accidents involving shift workers who have been deprived of adequate, restful sleep.

HEALTH FLASH

how much ATP our bodies produce. But many other factors also contribute to our energy experiences. For one thing, our very genes are believed to have unique "energy dispositions" encoded within them; to some degree, we seem to be born placid or wired. A number of hormones, neurotransmitters, and lifestyle factors also come into play to determine how alert we feel.

Here are the major energy boosters and zappers, which, once understood, can help us maximize that positive, ready-to-take-on-the-world feeling.

Keep an Eye on the Clock

Several factors that determine how much vitality we have are largely beyond our control. Perhaps the most significant of these influences is our endocrine system (see "The Hormone Factor" on page 104). Another is the fascinating inner device known as the biological clock.

The biological clock is not quite that mysterious mechanism women report as "kicking in" at a certain age and urging them to bear children. In fact, the biological clock is a circadian, or daily, pacemaker located inside the hypothalamus of both men and women. The internal biological clock coordinates the sleep/wake cycle, measuring day length independent of environmental cues. More important, the clock generates natural circadian rhythms that control fluctuations in body temperature, cardiovascular rate, and hormone secretions—all of which affect our energy levels.

Researchers have found that people experience natural alertness and sleepiness patterns that follow these inherent circadian rhythms. Both physical strength and mental alertness appear to be good in the morning and even better in the later afternoon hours, between 4:00 P.M. and 8:00 P.M.

Drowsier times of the day within the circadian cycle occur between 1:00 P.M. and 4:00 P.M.—regardless of preceding eating patterns—and around a person's regular bedtime. To anyone monitoring a baby's nap schedule or attending a 2:00 P.M. lecture, these troughs in alertness are already well-known. Europeans have all but structured their culture around them, observing leisurely afternoon siestas before returning to work in the early evening.

Because, like any biological process, the circadian system matures over time, adolescent and elderly energy patterns differ slightly from those in most adults. According to research done by Mary Carskadon, Ph.D., director of the sleep research laboratory at the E. P. Bradley Hospital of Brown University in Providence, Rhode Island, adolescents are virtually programmed to be owls, incapable of physical vigor and mental alertness until several hours after others. The reverse is true for the elderly, who become morning larks and need less sleep as their circadian systems age.

Recharge with Sleep

Sleep is crucial to energy and is something over which we usually have control. Most experts agree that the amount of sleep each of us needs to feel energized and ready to take on the day is personal—but on average, people need eight hours of sleep every night to feel rested. More universal are the symptoms we all display when we're short on sleep. If you require a five-alarm wake-up procedure, nod off during late afternoon drives, or fall asleep only minutes after reaching your bed, you are probably not getting enough sleep. Other less obvious signs that you are sleep-deprived include social withdrawal, frequent battles with minor health nuisances, reliance on caffeine to stay awake, and grumpy or irritable behavior.

According to Steven Reppert, Ph.D., director of the Laboratory of Developmental Chronobiology at Harvard Medical School, *when* you sleep is more crucial in determining your energy benefits than how much you sleep. Trying to sleep when it isn't dark out, for example, or delaying your sleep through travel to an earlier time zone, does not leave you properly rested; your body is too busy resisting the manipulation of its biological clock.

How you snooze is also critical in determining your energy level, says Margaret Moline, Ph.D., director of the Sleep/Wake Disorders Center at New York Hospital/Cornell Medical Center in New York City. She points out that many people spend a lot of time in bed and still miss out on sleep benefits. These low-energy people may suffer from sleep apnea, which affects about 2 percent of women. With this disorder, the sleeper stops breathing and snores in a way that repeatedly awakens her at night. Resting next to a snoring spouse or living on a busy street corner can also rob you of good shut-eye, which only occurs when your brain experiences both dreamy, R.E.M. sleep and deep, slow-wave sleep. If you wake too often, you never descend into deep sleep. Skipping or skimping on either sleep stage will cause you to awaken unrested. That is why drinking alcohol before bed, which disrupts the normal stages, can also leave you feeling enervated in the morning.

Eat to Energize

What we eat has a tremendous impact on our energy levels. In *Food and Mood: The Complete Guide to Eating Well and Feeling Your Best*, author and leading nutrition expert Elizabeth Somer, R.D., offers several helpful tips on how to maximize your energy levels through the foods you choose.

Eat a good breakfast. A morning meal is absolutely essential to supply you with daytime energy reserves and literally break the fast that you have sustained overnight. Eating a light, low-fat breakfast—light to avoid sluggishness and low-fat to save digestive energy—stimulates your metabolism and helps ensure that you will get an even supply of calories and nutrients throughout the day. (When you skip breakfast, you often overeat at night, not only bringing on unwanted weight gain but also causing a loss of good energy the next morning, when you feel full enough to skip breakfast again.) Try a meal rich in both carbohydrates and protein, such as low-fat vanilla yogurt with fruit, or orange juice and a toasted bagel topped with one tablespoon of peanut butter.

Drink caffeine only in moderation. Caffeine is a stimulant because it inhibits adenosine, a neurotransmitter in the brain that otherwise makes you tired. Drinking too much caffeine, however, can bring on an initial high chased by debilitating withdrawal symptoms, one of which is fatigue; you crave more caffeine to restore your energy and, in a vicious circle, only end up losing more energy. Caffeine depletes energy for two other reasons: It lingers in the body for three to four hours, making energy-restoring sleep elusive, and it is a diuretic, contributing to energy-sapping dehydration. Try to drink no more than 300 milligrams of caffeine (about three five-ounce cups of coffee) daily.

Drink twice as much water as you think you need. Mild dehydration is often the cause of feelings of fatigue or low energy, and it's easily prevented. In addition to regular fluids, you should be drinking at least six to eight eight-ounce glasses of water a day—even more than you feel thirsty for.

Get your carbohydrates from starch, not sugar. Carbohydrates from both sugar and starch are good energy sources because they contain glucose, the material needed to make ATP. Starchy foods, however, provide more sustainable energy because they release glucose into the blood slowly. Sugary foods dump glucose into the blood all at once, causing quick-reacting insulin secretions from the pancreas to rush in and move the excess sugar out. Blood sugar levels consequently drop dramatically and energy suddenly slumps again—sometimes to lower levels than before the sugar intake. While the sugar crash is less severe when buffered by other food, a diet with some protein and plenty of complex carbohydrates such as whole grains and fruit is a more reliable source of energy. Eliminating sugar altogether may be a good idea for clinically depressed people; in one study, patients' moods and energy levels improved after a few weeks without it.

Stay away from low-calorie diets. Eating less than 1,500 calories a day can slow down your metabolic rate by 30 percent and leave you seriously deficient of key energy-sustaining nutrients. On top of that, it can impair your memory, concentration, and judgment. If you are watching your weight, eating several small meals or well-balanced snacks in four-hour increments throughout the day is the best plan to keep your metabolism cranking and your energy sustained.

Eat a light lunch. While eating a midafternoon meal is important to rekindle your daytime energy, overdo it and you'll experience the Goldilocks effect. Foods rich in carbohydrates like pasta, bread, and most desserts are particular lunchtime no-nos if you can't afford to be yawning and spacing out at work. These foods raise your serotonin levels, inducing a post-meal drowsiness to which women are particularly sensitive. Eat a 500-calorie meal consisting of some carbs and more proteins like legumes, tuna, chicken, or low-fat dairy products. Proteins will boost your alertness and concentration and increase your tyrosine, an amino acid in the brain that enables dopamine and other energizing neurotransmitters to revitalize you.

Make sure you get enough iron. You don't have to be anemic to experience energy lows related to iron deficiency, according to several experts. If you are a committed daily exerciser who experiences heavy periods or uses an IUD, you should keep close track of your iron status. According to Somer, 80 percent of women who exercise vigorously are iron-deficient, since blood loss during menstruation doubles iron needs and exercise may exacerbate them, depleting iron reserves through sweat.

Women who have been pregnant within the last two years or who eat less than 2,500 calories a day are also apt to feel drained and irritable from iron loss. In order to meet the Daily Value for iron, which is 18 milligrams, women should be sure to eat iron-rich foods (the best are lean meats, beans, tofu, and Cream of Wheat cereal) and refrain from drinking coffee or tea with meals, which can flush out iron before it's absorbed. Do check your iron levels with a doctor before deciding to take iron supplements. "Women should be cautious about taking iron supplements without knowing their bodies and their own iron statuses," advises Kathleen Foell, director of health education at the Spence Center for Women's Health in Boston. "Too much iron can be damaging to your cells and may even contribute to heart disease."

Exercise for Energy

It's no secret that exercise is invigorating: It wakes up your nervous system, speeds up your metabolic rate, increases blood flow to your brain and muscles, and stimulates mood-elevating hormones. Also established is that exercise helps you go to sleep at night, over time producing the stamina for you to do and endure more without tiring. Thirty minutes of daily aerobic activity can up your energy level several notches. What's less well known is that strength training can significantly impact your energy.

In her book *Strong Women Stay Young*, Dr. Nelson shows that a particularly successful way for women to energize as they age is through basic strength training two to three days a week. Her principle is simple and supported by new research: The stronger you are, the easier it is to move and become more active. Though strength training is not aerobic, it does improve aerobic capacity and your physical desire to work out. Since half the battle of increasing your energy through exercise is rallying yourself to action, strength training really helps get you going.

In addition, aerobic exercise alone doesn't maintain the mass of your muscles, which house the ATP manufactured from glucose, Dr. Nelson points out. The use-it-or-lose-it rule applies here particularly to women, who at age 40 can expect to begin replacing up to one-half pound of muscle (and the ATP stocked inside) each year with fat. Strength training, however, reverses this process. As your muscles grow and become more active, the level of ATP increases, which makes you more energetic.

Revive Your Mental Energy

Sometimes, even when you're exercising regularly, sleeping well, and eating right, you still feel beat. Chances are that other factors such as overwhelming stress or grief are sapping your mental energy. While many of these negative external forces may be beyond your control, you can investigate your social life for more stoppable mental energy drains.

According to Susan Forward, Ph.D., a psychologist and author of *Emotional Blackmail*, the best way to minimize energy depletion of this sort is to develop self-protective antennae that identify the people, interactions, or events that make you feel guilty or inadequate. Then "you must empower yourself by working up the courage to confront and deal with your emotional drains," advises Dr. Forward. "Because nothing is more annoying than assuming a victim mentality and feeling helpless. The more proactive you are in your life, the more energy you are going to have."

This suggests perhaps that we should identify and recognize our individual energy sources—the people, ideas, and passionate pursuits that validate and inspire us—just as we should our energy drains. For, ultimately, our happiness has a lot more to do with how alive we feel than whether we chose the bagel or the chocolate doughnut at breakfast time.

The Hormone Factor

Six hormones play a major role in how energetic—or enervated—we feel. Here's a look at what they are and how they relate to our energy levels.

Estrogen. Responsible for many female sex characteristics as well as the regulation of the female cycle, the hormone estrogen is a mild antidepressant associated with a woman's sense of well-being. When lacking estrogen, many women feel forgetful, unable to concentrate, anxious, or low on initiative. Estrogen levels peak in the first two weeks of the menstrual cycle and diminish significantly in the last, after ovulation. Of course, estrogen production also falls dramatically with menopause.

Progesterone. This hormone, which prepares the lining of the uterus for pregnancy and also helps to regulate our cycles, is the one that makes us feel PMS-y—irritable, depressed, tired, and achy. In high levels, progesterone is thought to kill off sex drive, diminishing energy in part by suppressing dopamine, one of the neurotransmitters in the brain that keeps us motivated and mobilized for action. In contrast to estrogen levels, progesterone levels increase during the last two weeks of our menstrual cycles. They also peak when we are pregnant or nursing, making us feel tired and foggy-headed.

Women undergoing hormone replacement therapy must take progesterone as well as estrogen, since unopposed estrogen increases the risk of uterine cancer. But birth control pills use about six times as much progesterone as is used in hormone replacement therapy. Some hormone specialists find it surprising that such a vast number of women ask for birth control pills, considering progesterone's rather unappealing profile. "Unbeknownst to many," warns Theresa

Crenshaw, M.D., a sex therapist in San Diego and author of *The Alchemy of Love and Lust*, "progesterone is one of the most potent (libido-depressing) drugs around. It is likely to provide birth control by killing off your sex drive and lowering your energy level."

Other experts assure that progesterone poses no threat to your sexual energy, explaining that any problems presented by the progesterone in oral contraceptives are more likely to involve weight gain or mood change. Today progesterone has fewer side effects, they say, and only rarely is it prescribed by itself; varying amounts of estrogen usually buffer the progesterone in contraceptives. Clearly, anyone who considers taking estrogen and progesterone—for birth control or menopausal symptoms—needs to consult an experienced health practitioner and seek the balance that feels right to her.

Testosterone. Like estrogen, this hormone works as an antidepressant. Present in women but 20 to 40 times more prevalent in men, testosterone increases aggressive, self-confident, and energetic behavior and is the hormone behind sexual desire in both sexes. Interestingly, because male testosterone levels fluctuate daily in 15- to 20-minute cycles, men experience the equivalent of three "mini-periods" an hour! The energy that women derive from testosterone is more constant. For both sexes, exercising, sexual fantasizing, meat-eating, and the experience of winning produce energy from testosterone. Testosterone production decreases after menopause, and some doctors prescribe small doses of the synthetic hormone to older women to increase their zest and sex drive. There have been no long-term studies on the safety of these supplements.

Dehydroepiandrosterone (DHEA). Another key energy hormone with antidepressant effects, it is found in both sexes in equal proportions. DHEA energizes because it improves cognition, protects the immune system, and increases sex drive. According to Dr. Crenshaw, high DHEA levels crank up your metabolism, allowing you to eat normally and burn more fat. Because being lean actually raises your DHEA levels, lean people not only find it easier to lose weight but also feel more energetic. Sounds unfair, but it's just one more reason to work out. Puberty and pregnancy—as well as vigorous exercise, transcendental meditation, and other forms of stress reduction—can all contribute to increases in DHEA. You are likely to stunt your DHEA production when you drink alcohol, take oral contraceptives, display type A behavior, or encounter chronic illness or stress. DHEA supplements are not approved by the Food and Drug Administration and should be avoided: They may increase cancer risks in both women and men.

Thyroid hormone. The thyroid gland's hormonal system, which is primarily responsible for metabolism, can also greatly impact your energy levels. Many women—including 20 percent of those over 60—endure overwhelming fatigue, chilliness, weight gain, constipation, and muscle cramps, not realizing their thyroids are "hypo," or underactive. Unlike the more dramatic hyperthyroidism (which gets the thyroid working too hard, accelerating the heartbeat

Energy You Can Do Without

Not all energy is good: Your body can also produce energy that diminishes your sense of well-being.

Stress is one kind of troublesome energizer. When you experience a stress reaction, the involuntary rush of the fight-or-flight response raises your heart and respiratory rates, increases your blood pressure, and tenses up your muscles. The energy zoom you experience may be thrilling, but it is not sustainable. Surges of the stress hormone cortisol, which floods your bloodstream during a stress response, in fact decrease both your DHEA and testosterone levels. Over time, more severe stress can suppress your immune system and greatly tax your brain, often giving you problems with attention, concentration, and short-term memory.

Mania also provides great rushes of energy which, when expressed mildly, look like healthy high spirits. But mania is usually accompanied by incredible volatility and unreliability. You may be unable to carry out plans and ideas because you can't sit still or maintain one constant mood. During serious manic episodes, you might chatter incoherently, max out your credit cards, or act sexually uninhibited. Mania is a harmful mood disorder brought on by a chemical imbalance in the brain. If you or someone you know displays this kind of pathological, mental high gear, seek help.

and producing uncomfortable excess energy), hypothyroidism often goes undiscovered or misdiagnosed. To avoid this, expert endocrinologists recommend that all women over 35 take a yearly blood test for their thyroid hormone levels. Fortunately, when detected, hypothyroidism can be cured quite easily with small daily doses of a synthetic thyroid hormone.

Melatonin. Manufactured in the brain's pineal gland, melatonin is known as the youth hormone because some people believe that it boosts the immune system and delays aging. But its most important role is to make us drowsy and bring on energy-refurbishing sleep. Under normal conditions, melatonin levels rise with the darkness in the evening, heighten between midnight and 6:00 A.M., and promptly drop off when bright morning light hits the eye. On cloudy or dim winter days, production of the hormone continues, and your urge to stay snuggled in bed is strong. You have probably heard of melatonin supplements used to cure jet lag or insomnia. Taken only occasionally, they appear to be safe (check with your doctor first), but do not take them regularly. Their long-term effects are simply not known.

Melatonin levels peak during childhood and decline gradually after puberty, so that by the time we are 50 to 70 years old, we often have only trace amounts left. This explains in part why we sleep less as we age. Because of its unique role in the sleep/wake cycle, melatonin is the only known hormone that can be said to help govern the circadian rhythms, which run our biological clocks.

part three

The Weight You Want

Quick Quiz

What's Your Diet Personality?

Following is a list of questions that will help you customize your weight-loss program so that you'll take pounds off and keep them off. Every question has four different personality descriptions. Using the numbers 1 through 4, rank each set of descriptions from the one that describes you least (1) to the one that describes you best (4). Remember, each description gets a number, and you can use each number only once per question.

1. When it comes to new health information, I . . .

____A. read several different sources to make sure they are giving the same advice.

____B. like to see statistics and how the information was compiled before believing it.

____C. don't have time to read the news.

____D. like to try new things, especially if it has worked for someone else.

2. When I dress in the morning, I . . .

____A. wear what makes me feel good that day.

____B. first watch the Weather Channel before deciding what to wear.

____C. wear what I planned at the beginning of the week for that day.

____D. wear what fits my mood.

3. I grocery shop . . .

____A. when we're out of food, and I buy what looks good.

____B. by buying only what's on the list I compiled from my weekly menu.

____C. by compiling a list of what's on sale.

____D. without a list and buy what seems good for my body.

4. When I pass my favorite fast-food restaurant, I . . .

____A. stop if it's mealtime but check nutritional information first.

____B. almost always stop to get my favorite food, even if I'm not hungry.

____C. stop if it's mealtime and get my favorite food.

____D. stop only if I've planned it into my weekly meals.

5. When contemplating my weekend activities, I prefer . . .

_____A. to plan several days in advance.

_____B. intellectually stimulating activities.

_____C. to keep my options open until Friday.

_____D. activities that help my personal growth.

6. The household chore I like best is . . .

_____A. choosing newspaper and magazine subscriptions for my family.

_____B. organizing kitchen and bathroom cabinets.

_____C. finding activities to help everyone in my family grow personally.

_____D. decorating the house so that it's an enjoyable, fun place to live.

7. In relationships with others, I . . .

_____A. am sometimes late to planned activities because I get involved in something fun and forget the time.

_____B. am known to get impatient when I'm not understood.

_____C. am considered idealistic.

_____ D. often have expectations of how others should behave.

8. Those who know me well say I am . . .

_____A. reliable and dependable.

_____B. empathetic and inspirational.

_____C. fun to have around when things become dull.

_____ D. intelligent and clever.

9. If I'm trying to lose weight, I will . . .

_____A. plan my meals in the morning, following my guidelines.

_____B. ignore my food plan if I'm busy or it doesn't sound good to me.

_____C. plan meals weekly and eat what's on my plan, even if it doesn't sound good to me that day.

_____D. fix something healthy, but I don't necessarily follow a meal plan.

10. When it comes to filing taxes, I . . .

_____A. don't get to it until the very last minute.

_____B. save my receipts throughout the year, then file my taxes by January 15.

_____C. enter my financial information on a computer and then use it to fill out my tax forms.

_____D. would rather hire someone to do it.

Scoring

Transfer your answers to the table below. Note that the spaces for scoring are not always in A-B-C-D order. Then total your points in each column.

(continued)

1. _____A. _____B. _____C. _____D.
2. _____C. _____B. _____D. _____A.
3. _____B. _____C. _____A. _____D.
4. _____D. _____A. _____B. _____C.
5. _____A. _____B. _____C. _____D.
6. _____B. _____A. _____D. _____C.
7. _____D. _____B. _____A. _____C.
8. _____A. _____D. _____C. _____B.
9. _____C. _____A. _____B. _____D.
10. _____B. _____C. _____A. _____D.

_____ _____ _____ _____

What Your Type Means

Compare your scores for the four columns. Which one is highest? This is your diet personality. If two scores are nearly equal, read the descriptions for both personalities to see which fits you best.

❖ Highest score in column 1: organized
❖ Highest score in column 2: analytical
❖ Highest score in column 3: spontaneous
❖ Highest score in column 4: inspirational

Organized. You thrive on rules and schedules. Your kitchen cabinets are likely to be highly organized; everything has its place in your home. You're committed and usually prepared for anything. Your diet Rx:

❖ Plan a week or two of menus at a time to make shopping and cooking easier. Make big batches of favorite recipes and serve them throughout the week. (For more meal-planning strategies, see 101 Easiest Ways to Win at Weight Loss on page 118.)
❖ Check off what you've eaten. Food logs keep you in the organized groove you love. Consider counting calories or fat grams. (You can make short work of those calories by following the advice in No-Sweat Ways to Burn Calories All Day on page 139.)
❖ Be flexible. "What works for you the first month of dieting might not be your optimum strategy for the fifth month," says Susan J. Bartlett, Ph.D., associate director of clinical psychology at Johns Hopkins School of Medicine in Baltimore.

Analytical. You're an information-gatherer, approaching life as if it were a science, says Indiana-based personality consultant Charles Yokomoto, Ph.D. You enjoy complexity and problem-solving. Your diet Rx:

❖ Have fun finding new and different ways of meeting your nutrition goals. Try three meals a day with snacks or several mini-meals—whatever fits your lifestyle. (For more clever weight-loss ideas that work, turn to 101 Easiest Ways to Win at Weight Loss on page 118.)

❖ Challenge yourself. You love figuring out how to enjoy your favorite foods and still lose weight.

❖ Take action. Since you enjoy gathering information, you may get stuck in that stage.

Spontaneous. You live life as it comes, expanding each moment to over-flowing. You look for variety and maximum flexibility. You hate schedules and have a crisis approach to life. You're not much for rules, but if they're fun, interesting, and not too strict, you may follow them. Your diet Rx:

❖ Skip rigid food plans. If they don't fit into your lifestyle, you'll just ignore them.

❖ Keep problem foods out of the house. You'll eat them if the mood seizes you. (Stop Feeding Your Emotions on page 170 takes a closer look at mood-driven eating.) Similarly, change your route to work to avoid the doughnut store.

❖ Set short-term goals. For you, there's always tomorrow and the chance to start over. Daily goals, such as eating a piece of fruit with every meal, thwart your tendency to "do it later."

Inspirational. You're always interested in improving yourself, mentally and physically. People often confide in you because you're a great listener and you have a wonderfully kind, effective way of inspiring others. Your diet Rx:

❖ Stick with the basics: Eat right and exercise. You're easily enticed by new research—even if it's very preliminary—and by new weight-loss products. (For the truth about such weight-loss aids, see The Verdict on Diet Pills on page 128.)

❖ Patrol portions. You're likely to enjoy an extra helping of a food you love, so dish up just a single serving.

❖ Avoid negative influences. Criticism affects you more deeply than other personality types. Learn to draw on your inner strength. (And be sure to read Is Your Family Sabotaging Your Diet? on page 174.)

❖ Reward yourself frequently. Buy a new outfit, a motivational book, or perhaps a bread machine to make hearty and healthy whole-grain breads.

The Most Common Weight-Loss Questions Answered

I f you've stood in the mirror frowning at your hips, tummy, or thighs, or if you've consulted an "ideal body weight" chart and found that you're pounds away from perfect, then you have probably dreamed about how much weight you want to lose. You're not alone. By one estimate, two of every three women say they feel flabby and want to firm up. In fact, the desire to slim down is so pervasive in this country that we Americans spend more than $4 billion a year on weight-loss programs, fat substitutes, and diet drugs. That's right—*$4 billion.*

Such products have appeal because they promise a quick fix. And often they do work . . . for a while. But eventually, inevitably, the pounds creep on again.

The real key to permanent weight loss, experts say, is eating healthfully and exercising regularly. Yes, these strategies require more effort—but the lasting results are worth it.

Fat Facts and Fiction

No matter how savvy you may be about dieting and weight loss, there are probably plenty of questions you've never asked, but wish you had the answers to. Here they are.

Motivation

Matters

When it comes to pound-paring, the most important factor isn't diet or exercise. According to a new study from the University of Rochester in New York, the key to weight loss is (surprise, surprise) self-motivation.

When researchers tracked the weight-loss histories of 128 extremely overweight women and men, they found that folks pressured by friends or family members didn't keep the pounds off. Neither did folks who used guilt or humiliation to pressure themselves to lose. On the other hand, people who were self-motivated by reasons such as a healthier lifestyle were most likely to succeed—regardless of age, gender, or even how much they had to lose.

The bottom line? The best time to attempt weight loss is when you are truly ready—not when you're simply sick of being told you should. Where there's a will, there may be a way. But the will has to come from within.

How much weight can you deduct for clothing? It all depends on what you're wearing, of course, and whether your robe, for example, is thick terry cloth or gauzy silk. But the average weights of these items will give you an idea: medium-thickness terry cloth robe, 2 pounds, 9.1 ounces; flannel nightgown, 8.9 ounces; oversize T-shirt, 7.1 ounces; size 10 blue jeans, 1 pound, 9.4 ounces; moccasin slippers, 7.6 ounces; watch, 1.4 ounces; ring (thin gold band with stone), 0.2 ounce.

How much extra weight can you really attribute to being bloated just before your period? At the end of your monthly cycle, your body retains water just in case it needs to increase its blood volume to feed a pregnancy. But, according to Laurie R. Green, M.D., an obstetrician/gynecologist in San Francisco, the range of weight gain is only from about eight ounces to (in the case of extreme bloating) three pounds. Any other premenstrual pounds come from dietary changes (also known as PMS pig-outs).

What are some of the most destructive diets ever made popular? The variety is endless: all-meat or -carbohydrate or -liquid, mostly grapefruit, mostly hard-boiled eggs, to name a few. One even consisted of eating 14 pounds of grapes a day. "The weirder the diet, the more it captures public imagination," says Jeanne Goldberg, Ph.D., associate professor at the School of Nutrition Science and Policy at Tufts University in Boston. "These fad diets make a few people very rich, while a lot of other people get hurt."

Any diet that focuses on one food group at the expense of others is unhealthful, says Dr. Goldberg. The best diet? "Foods you can live with that are generous in complex carbohydrates, moderate in lean proteins, and light on fats," she advises. "Eat small portions and exercise. Forget the miracles."

Which dietary problems can you blame on your mother? Mom may share the "weight" with other people in your gene pool, since heredity does have an enormous influence on whether you're overweight. Studies of identical twins reared separately show that, despite different upbringings, these siblings have similar weight and body fat distribution 65 percent to 80 percent of the time, says Ronald Kleinman, M.D., chief of pediatric gastroenterology and nutrition at Massachusetts General Hospital in Boston.

Genetic destiny can be combated with self-control, though. "Genes only allow you to accumulate fat if you overeat or underexercise," says Dr. Kleinman. "The key is to eat just enough to match the energy that goes out."

With a beach vacation rapidly approaching, can you realistically lose five pounds in a month? Five pounds in a month is a reasonable goal; you must simply cut 625 calories out of your daily regimen, says John Foreyt, Ph.D., director of the Behavioral Medicine Research Center at Baylor College of Medicine in Houston. He recommends carving half that amount from your diet and adding enough daily exercise to cover the rest (a one-hour walk would do it). More to lose? Up to two pounds a week, no problem. More than that can create health risks.

Why are there times when you're religious about your diet and still don't lose weight? This situation can happen after someone has been dieting for a bit, says Kristine Clark, R.D., Ph.D., director of sports nutrition for the Center for Sports Medicine at Pennsylvania State University in University Park. Let's say someone weighing 150 pounds has been eating 1,500 calories a day and loses 20 pounds. Now she weighs 130 pounds, but she stops losing. Part of her problem is that she needs fewer calories to sustain her new, lighter body weight. To get back on the losing track, she needs to decrease her calories to about 1,300 a day or increase her exercise.

I've always had the impression that some mysterious alchemy converts a pound of chocolate into five pounds of body fat. What's the real damage? Whether the calories come from chocolate or carrots, every time you accumulate 3,500 extra ones, they turn into a pound of body fat. One pound of milk chocolate contains approximately 2,350 calories. So assuming they aren't needed for daily energy requirements, you could conceivably eat that pound of chocolate plus an additional 8-ounce Hershey bar before a pound shows up on your scale.

Can you speed up your metabolism? Your basal metabolic rate (that is, metabolism) is the amount of energy needed to maintain your body's normal operations from blood circulation to breathing, explains Ann Grandjean, Ed.D., director of the International Center for Sports Nutrition in Omaha, Nebraska. Lots of things will temporarily increase your metabolism: lack of sleep, hot or cold environments, even a fever. But, she admits, "the effect these increases have upon weight loss is pretty insignificant."

"The best way to increase your metabolism is to increase muscle mass," she says. Muscle requires more energy to maintain than fat. Two women may both weigh 135, but if one has 20 percent body fat and the other 25 percent, the first woman will burn more calories.

Why don't you ever seem to lose weight on top if you're large breasted, but it's the first place it vacates when you're flat as a board? Perception is part of why it seems as if you lose the most weight where you least need it, says Dr. Foreyt. When you have little to lose in a particular spot, small changes are more noticeable. When you have more to lose, the opposite is true.

Yet, studies suggest that the greater proportion of initial weight loss comes from the upper body, says James Hill, Ph.D., professor at the Center for Human Nutrition at the University of Colorado in Denver. "What part of the upper body it comes from, belly or breast, depends upon the individual," he says. "It would be great if we could predict or target the weight loss, but we don't really understand it yet."

If the calorie loss from one-half hour on the treadmill barely equals a scoop of ice cream, why not skip the ice cream and the trip to the gym? This question gets one thing right: It's good to cut back on fatty foods, says Dr. Clark. But don't cut out exercise along with it. "All the dieting in the world isn't going to shape a body the way we want to be shaped," she says. "Exercise gives a body the tone that makes it look better."

And like the Energizer Bunny, the benefits of that exercise session keep on going. Exercise's ability to reduce stress while increasing well-being and self-esteem is well-documented. "Exercise also raises your metabolism, so you burn off calories for a while even after you've finished your workout," Dr. Clark explains. "And the more you exercise, the more muscle you develop. Muscle tissue burns more calories than other types of tissue (like fat), even when at rest."

Is it better to eat before exercise so you can work off the calories, or afterward, while your metabolism is chugging at a higher rate? From a dieting perspective, "a calorie is a calorie no matter when you use it," says Dr. Grandjean. "The real issue is whether you take in more than you use over time."

From an exercise perspective, pick the time that makes you feel best during your workout. Some people get shaky if they work out on an empty stomach, while others feel sluggish exercising on a full one. According to Dr. Grandjean, "there is no physiological reason to wait until after you eat to do moderate exercise." But Daniel Kosich, Ph.D., a Denver exercise physiologist, cautions that if your pre-exercise blood sugar is too low, your performance may suffer.

"If I were handing out dieting advice," Dr. Grandjean says, "I'd say eat at the time when you'll eat less. If exercising makes you feel ravenous afterward, eat something before you start so you won't get so hungry."

Dr. Kosich agrees, but he also warns that during a vigorous workout, your muscles demand more blood flow, and if you've just eaten a big meal, your

Lose Weight, Stay Slim

You've heard the pessimistic view: Few people who lose weight actually keep it off. Now for the optimistic one. New research published in the *American Journal of Clinical Nutrition* says keeping weight off really isn't as tough as we think. Researchers from the University of Pittsburgh School of Medicine and the University of Colorado analyzed survey responses of 629 women and 155 men who maintained at least a 30-pound weight loss for five years or more. And these people said keeping the weight off was easier than losing it.

"It's nice to know that a lot of people have been successful," says Mary Lou Klem, Ph.D., senior research fellow at the University of Pittsburgh School of Medicine. "They are extremely happy and healthy. So it must not be a miserable process."

Maintaining weight loss does require effort, says Dr. Klem. You must continue the same habits you began when you were losing weight. You can't revert to a high-fat diet and low-exercise lifestyle.

Some secrets of the successful fat-fighters:

❖ They exercise off an average of 2,800 calories a week—the equivalent of 28 miles of running or walking.

❖ Though they do watch their fat and calorie intake, they never go hungry. Each day they usually eat three meals and two snacks.

❖ They weigh themselves often. "If there's a weight increase, they're going to catch it quickly. Then they only need to make moderate changes in eating or exercise to get back on track," says Dr. Klem.

---

stomach is also demanding more blood for digestion, so this "competition" for blood may result in cramps or discomfort. For a light, pre-workout snack, Dr. Kosich suggests a banana or an energy bar, which is high in carbohydrates and low in fat.

Why does cellulite go right to the thighs and butt rather than someplace innocuous like the earlobe? Cellulite is just a kind of fat, and fat distribution, if you haven't noticed, seems to rely upon gender. Men typically deposit it in the belly, while women get their deposits in the butt and thighs. "We wish we knew why fat goes where it goes," says Dr. Hill. "It may well be related to sex hormones."

Two fat facts fuel Dr. Hill's speculation. During lactation, the fat cells in a woman's lower body release more fat than at any other time of her life, suggesting that this fat is, in part, held in reserve for the energy needs of having children. Also, after menopause (and the decline of sexual hormone production), women often change weight-gain patterns and get bellies just like guys.

So does this mean we can blame fat thighs on the ability to bear children? Is this the reason we have more cellulite than men? Probably, says Dr. Foreyt. Extra body fat is evolution's insurance policy that provides all stages of childbearing with emergency energy stores. It may even provide physical protection from outside bumps and knocks. That's why women typically have 20 to 22 percent body fat, while men have only 16 percent.

Not to keep whining about men, but why can so many of them eat as much as they want without gaining any weight? It's easy to think that men are immune to weight gain when you're picking at a salad, and your beanpole male buddy is devouring a mountain of spaghetti carbonara. "Studies show, though, that there are just as many overweight men as women," says Dr. Hill.

Of course, men can eat more than women because they are larger and have more muscle mass, so they need more calories to maintain themselves. "That's why they seem to get more bang for their buck when dieting or exercising," says Dr. Hill. "As bigger people, they expend more energy. Some data suggest that men are generally less sedentary, so they use up more calories that way, too."

How much do breasts weigh? Obviously, you can't generalize between a 32AA and a 36D. But John Kral, M.D., professor of surgery at the State University of New York Health Science Center in Brooklyn, says breast tissue weighs approximately the same as water, so anyone so inclined can make her own calculations: Just line your best-fitting bra with a large plastic bag and pour in enough water to fill one bra cup to its top. Measure the water (one fluid ounce of water weighs one ounce) and multiply by two.

How much more does muscle really weigh than fat? If you had a glob of fat that weighed 1 pound, the same size chunk of muscle would weigh 1.22 pounds, about 22 percent more.

Is it true that you can eat certain foods in combination with each other to burn calories more efficiently? The short answer is no. The longer answer is, "this is a ridiculous notion that makes no biological sense," according to Dr. Goldberg. It is an intriguing idea that has sold a lot of books, she explains, but it goes against all our knowledge of body chemistry and digestion.

Why is cellulite so hard to lose? Two reasons: First, because it's hard to lose fat, period, and cellulite is a concentration of fat. And second, because heredity has been unkind to those of us with cellulite. Some women have firm fat on their thighs and butts. And some have the kind of fat that's laid down in a pattern that creates ripples under the skin (also known as cellulite). Any good diet and aerobic exercise program (from swimming to brisk walking) will help reduce overall body size. Short of cosmetic surgery, that's the best you can do.

They say sex uses up about 150 calories. How did they do the research? This oft-cited figure may be just an estimate. "I don't think the calorie requirements of sexual activity have ever really been measured," says Eric Ravussin, Ph.D., a visiting scientist in exercise physiology at the National Institutes of Health.

Could that estimate be accurate? Making a rough calculation by tripling the amount of energy an average woman uses at rest, Dr. Ravussin concludes that burning 150 calories is possible if sexual activity lasts an hour.

101 Easiest Ways to Win at Weight Loss

M̲ark Twain once said, "The only way to keep your health is to eat what you don't want, drink what you don't like, and do what you'd druther not." Sound a bit too true when it comes to your attempts to lose weight? Luckily, it doesn't have to be that bad. Just follow these tips from nutrition and weight-loss experts. And for some extra inspiration, you'll find "Here's What I Did" stories from women who have lost 30 pounds or more and kept it off for more than a year.

1. Remove the skin from chicken—but wait until after you've cooked it. According to the U.S. Department of Agriculture, it's worth the few extra grams of fat you'll get from the skin during cooking, since the skin increases the meat's flavor, moistness, and tenderness. Resist the urge to eat it, though: It adds six grams of fat and 100 calories to your serving of chicken—just what you don't need.

2. To keep yourself on track, practice visualization. Imagine yourself fit and trim.

Here's What I Did: "If you can actually visualize yourself as the person you want to be, you'll become that person," says Kathy Wilson, 47, who took off more than 100 pounds. "When I felt like I couldn't do this for one more minute, I slipped in a motivational tape. Step by step, it would walk me through a visualization exercise, so I could see myself as I wanted to be."

Want to keep a raging appetite under control? Slice up a banana . . . and sniff it. Research suggests that the aroma of certain foods can trick your brain into thinking your stomach is full.

In tests at Chicago's Smell and Taste Treatment and Research Foundation, 3,193 overweight volunteers lost an average of nearly five pounds a month when they sniffed essence of peppermint, banana, and green apple whenever they felt hungry. And get this: The weight loss occurred despite no changes in diet or exercise.

Say what?

Believe it. Appetite is controlled by the brain, not the stomach. "The brain may think, 'I've sniffed it; therefore I've eaten it,'" says Alan Hirsch, M.D., the foundation's director and the author of *Dr. Hirsch's Guide to Scentsational Weight Loss*.

Two easy ways to take advantage of this aromatic effect on appetite: Eat your meals hot (when more odor molecules escape from food), and sniff your food before you eat it.

3. Use the buddy system. According to research conducted at Purdue University in Lafayette, Indiana, women who teamed up with supportive partners lost as much as 30 percent more weight than other dieters.

4. Eat slowly. It takes about 20 minutes for the food you've eaten to enter your bloodstream as glucose and "turn off" those feelings of hunger.

5. Vary your exercise routine for maximum benefit. The more muscle groups you use, the more calories you'll burn.

6. Put a lid on fatty bottled salad dressings, which have 135 to 155 calories per two-tablespoon serving. Opt for an equal portion of fat-free dressing, which has 30 to 50 calories per serving.

7. Lift weights. A pound of muscle burns about 35 calories a day when at rest, while the same amount of fat uses only 2 calories a day.

Here's What I Did: "It wasn't until I put on more muscle through resistance training that I was able to keep the weight off almost effortlessly," says Verona Mucci-Hurlburt, 37, who went from a size 18 to an 8.

8. Divide your dinner into courses. Have a cup of soup early, eat the main course with your family, and save dessert for a few hours later.

9. Don't skip meals. Eating throughout the day burns more calories because it increases your body's metabolic rate, which speeds up your fuel burning and, therefore, your fat burning.

10. Add a little zing to your life. Spicy meals can raise your metabolism, and eating them makes you burn slightly more calories than you would after downing blander fare.

11. Cut back on caffeinated coffee. Try a decaf cappuccino or, as a way to cut out calories, try water with a twist of lemon.

12. Follow the "eat to live," not "live to eat" rule. Use food as a fuel to keep moving instead of a way to enjoy get-togethers.

13. Drink lots of water. Water fills you up (without adding sodium or sugar to your system) and flushes toxins from your body.

Here's What I Did: "Drinking lots of water keeps me from snacking when I'm not hungry, and it gives me more energy," says Therese Revitt, 42, who lost 80 pounds and has run a marathon. "It also stopped what I thought were hunger headaches, which were probably due to dehydration."

14. Forget slipups. Everyone has days of overeating. Give the guilt a rest and focus on getting back on track.

15. To prevent overeating, snack more—on fresh fruits and vegetables, that is.

16. Say no to seconds, at first. If after 20 minutes you're still hungry, have a piece of fruit.

17. Eat a vegetarian meal once or twice a week.

18. If stress makes you head for food, try deep breathing or take a quick walk until the urge passes.

Here's What I Did: Call a friend. "I had to be willing to call my support people at 9 o'clock on a Friday night," says Barbara, 46, who's kept off 46 pounds for more than 15 years.

19. Schedule three 10-minute mini-workouts a day—aside from your regular exercise routine. They'll keep your metabolism up, reenergize you, and help keep cravings (and even stress) at bay.

20. Don't think "diet." Making healthy choices is a new way to eat—for life.

Here's What I Did: "I learned how to eat and live with it for the rest of my life," says Barbara Miltenberger, 42, who lost more than 40 pounds and hasn't seen any come back in three years.

"The best thing that I did was quit dieting," says Amy Reed. "I'd always find ways to cheat. So instead, I stopped forbidding myself certain foods and just started eating less of them." Reed, 36, has kept off more than 80 pounds for 13 years.

"Before I'd go to bed, I'd ask myself, 'Is what I did today something I could do for the rest of my life?' If I felt deprived, I'd do it differently the next day. If I thought, 'Yeah, I could do this again tomorrow,' then I was on the right track," says Revitt.

21. Avoid alcohol. It's high in calories, it stimulates your appetite, and it has a disinhibiting effect that can lead to overeating.

22. Change your traditional proportion of meat to vegetables: less of the for-

mer, more of the latter. You'll have less fat and fewer calories on your plate—and in your belly.

Here's What I Did: "I've been known to eat a whole bag of frozen vegetables, and with only a quarter-cup of pasta or stir-fry sauce, it's only about three grams of fat," says Mucci-Hurlburt. "It's saved my butt many times when I was really hungry and had to eat now."

23. If you have an urge to snack, brush your teeth.

Here's What I Did: Putting a note reading "Stop" on the refrigerator kept Reed from raiding it. Underneath she listed other things to do, like "Take a drink of water" and questions such as "Are you really hungry?"

24. Use light mayonnaise instead of regular and save nearly 100 calories per sandwich.

25. Learn what sets you bingeing and avoid those situations. If a late lunch always means you overeat, try to eat early (or at least have a healthy snack) on days when you know your noon break may be delayed.

26. When you're tempted to eat something that's unhealthful, ask yourself, "Is it worth having to walk for an extra half-hour?" The answer is usually no. If the answer is yes, be sure you include the extra time in your next walk.

27. When dining out, don't be afraid to ask that food be prepared the way you want it, such as without oil or butter. And always ask that sauces and salad dressings be served on the side so that you can control your intake.

Here's What I Did: "I'm not afraid to ask for dishes to be prepared differently," says Victoria Bennett, 39, who shed 60 pounds and has kept them off for five years. "My philosophy is that every restaurant has a grill and an oven. They don't have to fry everything."

28. To make your portions seem larger, eat off salad plates instead of dinner plates. You won't be tempted to load on more than you should—because there won't be room.

29. Don't weigh yourself. The scale doesn't give you realistic feedback because you gain muscle when you exercise, so you may gain pounds even though you've lost fat.

30. Set realistic goals. Trying to lose more than 25 pounds in two months is a recipe for failure. Talk with your doctor if you're not sure what your weight-loss time frame should be.

Here's What I Did: "My first goal was to lose only 10 pounds," says Rebecca, 46. "I had very high blood pressure, and my doctor said if I would just lose 10 pounds, he believed that I could get off the pills. Every other doctor before said I had to lose 100 pounds, and I thought 'I can't do that.' But 10 pounds . . . I thought, 'Maybe I can do that.' Doing it one bite at a time made it more achievable for me."

31. Stop eating when you're full, even if you still have food on your plate. Doggie-bag it if you don't want to waste it.

Here's What I Did: Better yet, don't wait to doggie-bag. "As soon as the server puts the food down in front of me, I cut the whole portion in half, put it on my butter plate, and ask her to wrap it," says Revitt. If you wait until the end of your meal, often you pick at it until the server returns.

32. Don't be discouraged by slow weight loss. Focus on the positive changes you've made and how much healthier you are.

Here's What I Did: "It took me a year to lose 100 pounds this time," says Rebecca, who has kept it off for eight years. "I had lost 100 pounds twice before, in less than six months each time, but I didn't maintain it."

33. Don't taste-test food while preparing it. The habit of sampling can add lots of unnecessary calories to your daily count.

34. Eat more soup. Broth-based, vegetable-laden soups are naturally low in fat and calories, and they're filling enough to be main dishes.

35. On special occasions, have either a dessert or an appetizer, but not both.

36. Keep your tastebuds titillated by trying new low-fat dishes.

37. Don't eat foods you don't like—even nutritious ones. Forcing yourself to eat something you hate may turn you off completely to healthy eating.

38. Reward your efforts, but not with food. Opt for a long bath or a new hairstyle.

39. Cravings often pass, so wait 30 minutes before giving in to that piece of cream pie. If you must, take one bite, and if it's not a 10 on the taste scale, don't finish it. Why waste calories on mediocre food?

Here's What I Did: "If I'm going to blow 500 or 600 calories, I want to make sure that I'm enjoying it to the max," says Mucci-Hurlburt. "Often, desserts look much better than they taste. If it tastes like cardboard, forget it. It's not worth it."

40. Buy fresh fruits and vegetables instead of canned. This will cut down on your intake of calories, sodium, and additives, plus the foods will taste better.

41. Don't have dessert on an empty stomach—be sure to eat a healthy meal first. That way, you'll be satisfied with a smaller slice, dish, or scoop.

42. Rev up your workout with red. A study at the University of Texas Medical Branch in Galveston suggests that red light may boost your energy and muscle strength. Try trading the white bulb in the lamp beside your stationary bike for a ruby one.

43. Don't try to lose weight for a special occasion. Wanting to drop 10 pounds before a vacation doesn't foster the kind of lasting commitment you need to make.

44. Share any high-fat food gifts you receive. (This is one case where re-gifting isn't rude—it's a survival skill.)

45. Prepare and freeze low-fat dishes in meal-size portions. Thaw one at a time to keep yourself from splurging.

46. Use applesauce in place of some or all of the oil or margarine in muffins, breads, stuffings, and cakes. Experiment until you're satisfied with the taste and texture.

47. Avoid sugar. Hungry for something sweet? Eat fruit. It's a powerhouse of vitamins, minerals, and fiber, with few calories and virtually no fat.

48. Buy "select" grades of meat, which are leaner than "prime" or "choice."

49. Don't eat after 7:00 P.M. Your body reaches peak metabolism about four hours after you've eaten, so if you eat shortly before bedtime, the food will more likely be stored as fat.

50. Reduce or eliminate butter whenever possible. Every tablespoon has 100 calories and 11 grams of fat.

51. Eat bigger servings—of the right foods. For example, have a large glass of orange juice instead of a small one. The extra calories are minimal, and you'll be getting two servings in one glass.

52. Take the stairs, not the elevator, whenever possible.

53. Watch those serving sizes. Just because food is low-fat or fat-free doesn't mean you can eat all you want. Calories do count, and they add up quickly.

Here's What I Did: "I stopped making six or seven grilled chicken breasts and thinking that everybody had to have two or three," Bennett says. "Now I make just one for each person."

54. Vow to watch TV only when exercising.

55. Don't bring home junk food or candy. If it's not there, you can't eat it.

Here's What I Did: "It's easier to fill the house with treats for my kids if I choose ones that I don't like, such as Oreo cookies," says 30-year-old Tammy Hansen, who trimmed off 60 pounds.

56. Curb your appetite at mealtimes by drinking a large glass of water beforehand.

57. Eat enough fiber. Because soluble fiber is a filler, it satisfies your appetite and provides you with lasting energy. Your goal should be 25 to 30 grams a day.

58. Read labels when shopping for food. Keep a running list of foods you've determined to be low-fat and low-calorie, and make them regulars in your diet.

59. Avoid anything with the words *breaded, scalloped, crispy, gravy, fried, au gratin, creamy,* or *flaky* on the label—that is, unless the calorie and fat counts show that the food is low-calorie and low-fat (deriving less than 30 percent of its total calories from fat).

Lose Weight—Without Pesky Exercise

A glass of cold water will frequently help silence your stomach until your next meal. But eight pints (128 ounces) of ice water a day may actually help you shrink that belly. According to Ellington Darden, Ph.D., author of *A Flat Stomach ASAP*, your body will expend 123 calories of body heat a day to warm that much ice water (at 40°F) to 98.6°F. As a result, you'll drop about a pound a month, and that doesn't even take into account all those calories you'll burn sprinting to the bathroom.

60. Keep a food diary. You'll be less likely to overeat or make bad choices when you have to write things down. Record every morsel of food that passes your lips.

Here's What I Did: "When I started keeping a food diary, I discovered that I was eating somewhere between 3,000 and 4,000 calories a day," says Rebecca, who found the number shocking.

61. Don't "diet." Drastically cutting your calories makes your body go into starvation mode to conserve energy, which slows your metabolism.

Here's What I Did: "As soon as I saw the weight coming off, I thought, 'If it's working at this rate, I'll try eating less so I'll lose more,'" admits Miltenberger.

"Then I'd stall or even put weight on because I was undereating and my metabolism slowed. I'd start losing again when I'd eat a little bit more," she says.

62. Recognize hunger differences. Learn to distinguish between a mental craving and a hungry stomach.

63. Get plenty of Zzzs. According to the Sleep Disorders Center at Emory University Medical Center in Atlanta, some studies show that when people don't get enough sleep, they eat more.

64. Avoid salt, which causes dehydration and bloating. Flavor your food with a variety of fresh herbs and spices.

65. To avoid buying sugary or high-fat snacks, never shop when you're hungry.

66. For lasting results, make a few small changes at a time. Switch from whole milk to 2 percent, and then to skim.

67. Instead of meeting friends for dinner, take them inline skating, to the gym, or for a walk.

Here's What I Did: When Reed finally succeeded in losing weight, her fiancé was a big help. "We didn't focus all our socializing around food. We went bike riding a lot and played tennis instead of going for pizza."

68. Play slow, calming music while you eat. A fast beat may make you eat faster, and possibly more.

69. Use a microwave, which preserves up to 100 percent more nutrients than a conventional stove.

70. Roasting meat in a pan allows it to soak up fat. Place a rack under the meat so the fat drips off during cooking.

71. Don't exercise on an empty stomach, which causes your metabolism to plummet. Doing so causes you to burn fewer calories during and after your workout.

72. Eat everything with a fork. Think about it: How many potato chips or cookies can you eat with a fork?

73. Don't give in to the "I blew it" feeling if you have a meal that's richer than usual. Just make sure to eat healthfully for the next three meals, and it'll all balance out.

74. Vary your meals to avoid feeling bored or deprived.

Here's What I Did: For variety, Helen Fitzgerald cooks rice, beans, and other grains in different liquids, such as tomato juice, apple juice, and beef or chicken stock. "Rice done in pineapple juice is especially good for rice puddings and Chinese dishes," she says. Fitzgerald, 61, has lost 51 pounds, and her husband has lost more than 150 pounds.

75. When you order a dessert at a restaurant, split it with someone else.

76. Don't grab something to eat on the run. Plan your meals in advance.

77. Don't wait until you're ravenous to eat. The hungrier you are, the harder it is to resist high-fat, high-calorie foods.

78. Avoid the yo-yo factor. Losing weight, putting it back on, and then losing it again is discouraging—and not healthy.

79. With the exception of raw fruits and vegetables, avoid finger foods. They're usually bad news, fat-wise.

80. Make weight loss a priority. Set aside time each week to exercise and create meal plans.

Here's What I Did: The beds might not get made, but Reed still makes time for exercise. "I have to schedule it in and let go of other things, like a perfectly clean house," she says.

81. Refrigerate homemade soups and stews for a few hours before eating, so that fat rises to the top and can be skimmed off.

82. Take a 30-minute walk after a big meal. You'll feel more alert and burn calories more quickly than if you rest.

83. Don't save up the day's calories for one meal—you'll only set yourself up for a binge situation.

84. Write down your emotional-eating triggers: stress, anger, loneliness, and so on. When this "head hunger" strikes, get busy with an activity instead, such as cleaning or jogging.

85. Use cooking sprays instead of oil or butter.

86. Divide your daily calorie intake into quarters—one for each meal, and one set aside for snacks. This keeps your metabolism high and prevents you from eating too many calories later in the day, when they're harder to burn off.

87. Don't think of anything as a forbidden food. Any food is okay as long as it's eaten in moderation—which means once a week, not once a day.

Here's What I Did: "If I want a piece of cake, I'll have one," says Debra Mazda, 44, who's 135 pounds slimmer than she was 13 years ago. "Then I just won't have another one for a week or so. Knowing that I can eat something and no one's going to say, 'You can't' works for me."

88. Don't arrive anywhere starving. Curb your appetite with a healthy snack before going to a party or out to dinner.

89. Don't crash-diet. You'll lose mostly water and muscle, and once you start eating again, you'll put the pounds right back on.

90. Discuss your goals with a trusted friend or family member. Sharing your commitment with another person may help you keep it.

Here's What I Did: "I started my first women's group when I first began exercising. It was just a bunch of women who got together once a week, and we would compare notes," says Mazda.

91. Don't eat in front of the TV, in bed, or while standing. Maintain one place in your home as the area where you eat.

Here's What I Did: "Even when I wanted potato chips, I set the table just as if I was going to sit down for a full-course meal," says Wilson. "I'd put a handful of chips on the plate, put the bag away, and then sit down to eat. I never just stand at the counter and eat now."

92. Stuff sandwiches with lettuce, tomatoes, onions, and other vegetables instead of meat and cheese.

93. Avoid prepackaged foods since they're typically high in calories and fat.

94. Dine at about the same time every day. This will get your appetite on track so you'll recognize true hunger more easily.

95. Use nonfat plain yogurt as a substitute for sour cream in casseroles, sauces, and dips.

96. Practice mindful eating so you'll appreciate the experience of dining. Taste and savor every bite.

Here's What I Did: If you just can't pass on some high-fat favorites, stick to the most flavorful ones. "A single slice of bacon is enough to flavor eggs or a potato," says Fitzgerald.

97. Fat-free labels make some foods seem healthier than they are. You're better off eating foods that are naturally low in fat and calories—like fruits and vegetables—instead of processed low-fat candies, pastries, and the like.

98. Find alternatives. You can even enjoy chocolate and still keep your waistline.

Here's What I Did: Bennett makes herself fat-free chocolate pudding with skim milk.

For Sarah, who lost 40 pounds and has kept it off for two years, a cup of sugar-free hot cocoa (about 20 calories), topped with a little fat-free whipped cream, does the trick.

99. To increase your activity level and get the exercise you need, find a passion.

Here's What I Did: "I have a dance background, and when I found jazzercise, I said, 'Thank God.' If somebody told me I had to go out and run five days a week, I'd still weigh 185 pounds," says Anne Geren, 41, who lost 55 pounds and has kept it off for 13 years.

100. Don't give up.

Here's What I Did: "There have been plenty of times when I've wanted to give up, but I didn't," says Mazda. "I realized a long time ago that entrepreneurs fall and rise up every time they lose a venture, but they just keep getting up." The same is true for weight loss.

101. For lasting results, aim for slow weight loss. If you lose a half-pound to a pound a week, you'll be 50 pounds lighter in a year.

16

The Verdict on Diet Pills

Millions of overweight Americans saw fen-phen and dexfenfluramine (Redux) as magic bullets. But for as many as one in three people, the diet pills were silent time bombs, slowly eating away at their hearts. Now that the drugs have been pulled off the market, what alternatives are available for women who want to slim down?

There's always the traditional approach: Reduce your intake of fat and calories, and exercise regularly. But if you've tried that and you still can't seem to shed those last few pounds—or if you're severely overweight—you may find some help in your nearest pharmacy or health food store.

In the pages that follow, you'll learn about the newest pharmaceuticals and herbal preparations that promise to give you an edge in the battle of the bulge. And you'll find out what to do if diet pills aren't for you.

Sibutramine: When Health Is at Stake

Among the latest entries in the diet pill sweepstakes is the drug sibutramine (Meridia). It's serious stuff. Sibutramine has been approved by the Food and Drug Administration for the treatment of serious obesity, usually accompanied by other health problems such as diabetes. (Serious obesity is defined as a body

Be Fruitful and Subtract Pounds

Researchers at the U.S. Army Academy of Health Sciences, on the grounds of Fort Sam Houston, Texas, have identified a natural substance that may turn out to be one of the most potent appetite suppressants around. The substance, a complex carbohydrate called pectin, is found in abundance in grapefruit, oranges, apples, and many other fruits.

The researchers asked 74 men and women to limit their breakfasts on two mornings to two glasses of orange juice. Half of the volunteers drank juice spiked with 5 to 20 grams of apple pectin. Over the course of four hours, those who consumed the pectin felt fuller than those who didn't. By lunchtime, the pectin group reported feeling moderately hungry, while the group that drank plain orange juice felt positively famished.

Apparently, pectin, which the body doesn't absorb, delays emptying of the stomach. This could explain its appetite-blunting effect, says James J. Cerda, M.D., a pectin expert at the University of Florida College of Medicine in Gainesville. As a bonus, pectin lowers cholesterol nearly as effectively as drugs do.

The Army study was too small to suggest an ideal dose of pectin. If you're interested in experimenting, you can order pure pectin powder from health food stores to mix into liquid. But drink fast: Pectin quickly turns juice into jelly. (The pectin sold for making jam is full of calorie-adding sugar.)

mass index of 30 or above, or 27 or above when accompanied by complicating factors.)

Sibutramine's effects depend upon your situation. Studies have shown that the drug can bolster weight loss by 5 to 10 percent. So a person who loses, say, 50 pounds may get a 5-pound "bonus" when taking sibutramine. The difference isn't as substantial as it would have been with fen-phen, according to Robert H. Eckel, M.D., vice-chairman of the nutrition committee of the American Heart Association. But in exchange, sibutramine may provide some significant benefits to those with obesity-related health problems.

Of course, for sibutramine to work, you still have to do your part. The drug's benefits were documented in people who were also dieting and exercising. "Diet and exercise should still be a major part of the equation," Dr. Eckel advises.

Complications may develop. Research has found that some people with high blood pressure saw their readings climb even higher while taking sibutramine.

If you already have high blood pressure, Dr. Eckel says, either you shouldn't take this drug or your blood pressure should be monitored very carefully during the first few weeks.

The bottom line? Sibutramine is for only those folks who really need it. Ask your doctor whether it's right for you.

Orlistat: Zaps Fat at Its Source

Another prescription fat-fighter, orlistat (Xenical), is still awaiting the Food and Drug Administration's approval. Orlistat works by preventing your body from absorbing about one-third of the fat you consume.

If you're already moderating your fat intake, orlistat could help you lose weight or keep off the weight you've lost, according to Judith Stern, R.D., Sc.D., professor of nutrition and internal medicine at the University of California, Davis. For example, the first clinical study of orlistat found that people who used the drug and ate a low-fat, reduced-calorie diet lost an extra five pounds, on average, compared with dieters not using the drug. That's not an excuse to stop exercising, though. "You also have to try to modify your lifestyle," she says.

Of course, your body has to get rid of that unabsorbed dietary fat somehow. That's why some people who take orlistat (especially those whose diets are high in fat) may experience diarrhea and abdominal cramping. Orlistat can also interfere with your body's absorption of vitamins D and E and beta-carotene. So anyone who takes the drug should talk to her doctor about how to make up for the nutrients that she's losing.

Like sibutramine and any other prescription weight-loss medication, orlistat is not for casual or cosmetic use. It is appropriate only for those whose weight is putting them at risk for other health problems.

Herbs: Slimming Aids from Nature

Because weight-loss medications are generally recommended only for people with serious weight problems, and because the medications can have side effects, many women are choosing an alternative route to slimness. As a result, "natural" diet aids have become a nearly $30-billion-a-year industry. These herbal preparations promise to take off the pounds safely and effectively. The question is, do they really work?

Herbs can promote weight loss in four primary ways. They can speed up your metabolism, flush waste and water from your system, dull your appetite, or dampen your tastebuds. But you have to know what you're doing to use an herbal product properly.

Here's the lowdown on each type of herbal diet aid.

Herbs that rev up your metabolism. It's an age-old story: While some people stay slender no matter how much pizza they inhale, others seem to put on weight just by thinking about a slice. The culprit? Could be a sluggish metabolism. The solution? Speed it up, of course.

Enter metabolism-boosting herbal diet aids. These products crank up your body's calorie-burning mechanism by way of nervous system stimulants such as ephedrine (from the herb ephedra) and caffeine. But while they may manipulate your metabolism slightly, what these products mainly do is signal your adrenal glands to pump out more of the hormone adrenaline, causing you to become somewhat hyper and edgy. You may shed a few pounds because you're more active, but eventually, your extra energy will turn into stress and nervousness.

Continual use of this combination of metabolism-boosting herbs (such as ephedra) and caffeine (found in herbs such as kola nut, maté, guarana, and camellia) simply isn't smart. In fact, it's downright risky. When you take any of these products frequently and in large doses (what's considered a large dose would depend on the product), you risk experiencing side effects such as agitation and insomnia. You're also in danger of developing high blood pressure or even having a heart attack. So steering clear is best.

A simple, healthful way to speed up your metabolism is to eat Chinese, Thai, or other foods flavored with hot peppers and spicy mustard. Researchers at Oxford Polytechnic in England attribute this metabolic boost to what's called the diet-induced thermic effect. Simply put, eating hot spices triggers an increase in calorie burn. In the study, 12 people consumed one of two meals. The meals were identical, except one included about one-half teaspoon each of red pepper and mustard sauce. Eating that one teaspoon of hot seasonings temporarily increased people's metabolic rates an average of about 25 percent.

Herbs that flush out your system. When used carefully by following the package directions and the advice of health care professionals, herbal laxatives (such as senna, cascara sagrada, and aloe powder) and herbal diuretics (such as dandelion, juniper, uva ursi, and parsley) are good natural medicines. When sold as weight-loss formulas . . . well, that's another story. Sure, taking any of these herbs alone or in combination may over time cause you to drop a couple pounds of fluid and bulk through repeated bathroom visits. But such weight-loss tactics certainly aren't healthy or safe.

Why? Because along with water and waste, herbal laxatives and diuretics flush important vitamins and minerals from your body. Using laxatives continually can create a dependency. And diuretics can overwork your kidneys, causing mineral imbalances that leave you weak and light-headed. Eventually, the imbalances and dehydration caused by these products can even lead to heart failure.

The bottom line is to stay away from any product promising to flush away pounds. And if you have a problem with water retention, consult your doctor before trying to relieve it with any type of diuretic product. This condition can signal a serious problem, such as heart disease.

A better bet is to shake the salt habit. Okay, you know that a high salt intake makes you retain water, so you shelve the shaker while trying to drop pounds. But you may not have thought to steer clear of prepared foods that are high in sodium. Some baddies: Store-bought baked goods, sausage, lunchmeats, hot dogs, canned vegetables (except those with no salt added), potato chips, pickles, olives, Parmesan and Cheddar cheeses, canned soup (except low-sodium varieties), and nuts (except unsalted varieties).

Herbs that curb your appetite. Sure, you've heard it a gazillion times: The safest and most effective way to lose weight is to eat less. Of course, if it were that easy, we'd all be eating less and losing all kinds of weight, right? Well, good news: Research has shown that certain herbs—such as guar gum seeds, glucomannan, and *Garcinia* (also known as brindal berry or tamarind)—can help you safely curb your appetite.

Some of these herbs work by absorbing water in your stomach and expanding into bulk that fills you with empty calories. Glucomannan (derived from the herb konjak), for example, absorbs an amazing 50 to 200 times its weight in water.

The herb *Garcinia*, on the other hand, works by altering the way your body metabolizes sugar. One study showed that overweight people who took the herb for two months ate about 10 percent less during meals and ultimately dropped an average of 11 pounds. Combine any of these appetite-suppressing herbs with a healthy diet and exercise, and of course, the weight-loss rewards multiply.

How much of these appetite-suppressing herbs should you take? Pills, capsule sizes, and concentrations vary from one product to the next, so follow the package directions closely. Generally, experts suggest trying 350 to 600 milligrams with about eight ounces of water.

Herbs that work by scent. Just walking by a bakery can start your stomach growling. But research has shown that getting a whiff of certain other aromas may actually help keep your appetite at bay. According to neurologist Alan Hirsch, M.D., director of the Smell and Taste Treatment and Research Foundation in Chicago, certain food smells trick your brain into thinking you've already eaten, thereby helping you cut calories and lose weight.

In his research, Dr. Hirsch tracked more than 3,000 middle-aged women who weighed about 200 pounds. The women sniffed peppermint, apple, and banana scents whenever they felt hungry. On average, they shed about 30 pounds in six months without a special diet or exercise program. In fact, the more they sniffed, the more they lost.

Several aromatherapy companies offer a number of herbal diet aids containing slimming scents. Some come as essential oils that you heat in a potpourri cooker (you put in a few drops with a certain amount of water), drop on a lightbulb ring (which sits on top of the bulb and releases the scent when it heats up), or add to your bath before you climb in. You can also buy a similarly scented bath or shower gel.

There Is Another Way

Maybe herbal diet aids haven't worked for you. Or maybe you're concerned about the safety of prescription weight-loss drugs. Don't give up your hopes of slimming down. Just follow the proven advice of diet doctors.

First, don't give up, Dr. Stern says. You can't postpone your weight-loss efforts until the next miracle pill comes along. "Obesity kills, just not overnight," she notes.

Second, realize that you don't need pills to shed pounds. People who use diet aids tend to credit the pills with their weight-loss success. What they need to realize is that if they lost weight, they did it themselves, says Gerard J. Musante, Ph.D., director of Structure House Center for Weight Control and Lifestyle Change in Durham, North Carolina. Most important, they have to believe that they can continue to lose weight without help from drugs or pills.

"Soon, you'll realize that you can do this yourself every day, every week, every month," says Beverly A. Enos, a spokesperson for the weight-loss support group TOPS (Take Off Pounds Sensibly). She shed 70 pounds more than 20 years ago without diet aids—and she has kept them off.

By exercising more and monitoring what you eat—strategies that have proven successful for millions of people—you, too, can succeed.

17

Do I Have to Exercise?

B y now, most everyone knows that exercise is an essential component of any weight-loss program. Of course, that doesn't necessarily provide enough motivation to get off one's duff and *do* something.

The fact is that many women don't like to work out—at least not at first, when the effort seems to far outweigh the results. Eventually, exercise gets easier. You'll even look forward to slipping into your workout clothes and working up a sweat for 30 minutes or so.

But if you're still at that "Do I have to?" stage, you may welcome this news. Yes, you really should work out, but you don't have to train like a triathlete to get results. How long and how hard you go at it really depends on what you hope to achieve, says James Rippe, M.D., director of the Center for Clinical and Lifestyle Research in Shrewsbury, Massachusetts.

With that in mind, here are some basic guidelines that are tailored to specific fitness goals.

If You Want to Slim Down . . .

"The notion of 'no pain, no gain' is outdated," notes Larry Durstine, Ph.D., director of clinical exercise programs at the University of South Carolina in

Take a Shortcut to Fitness

Many women are reluctant to engage in strength training because they think it's too inconvenient and time-consuming. Yet new research suggests that you don't need to work out as often or as long as previously thought to reap the benefits.

In the largest study of its kind so far, Wayne Westcott, Ph.D., strength consultant to the YMCA of the United States of America, examined the relationship between strength training and body composition in more than 1,000 people. He and his colleagues found that twice-a-week sessions produced 90 percent as much benefit as three-times-a-week sessions in terms of muscle gain and fat loss. "That's what most middle-aged and senior adults we train are interested in—'How do I look? What's my muscle gain and fat loss?'" says Dr. Westcott.

In a similar study, researchers at the Center for Exercise Science at the University of Florida in Gainesville considered whether the number of sets per session influences the effectiveness of strength training. (A set consists of a specific number of repetitions of an exercise.) The researchers found that over the course of 14 weeks, one set produced exactly the same benefits as three sets in people who were just beginning strength training.

When Dr. Westcott set out to determine the number of sets necessary for fitness, he discovered that people who were doing only one set of 10 repetitions per exercise gained about 2½ pounds of muscle and lost about 4½ pounds of fat in two months. "This is the way to go if you're just starting out or if you're limited on time," he says.

The pared-down minimum won't turn you into Arnold Schwarzenegger. But it will build muscle, reduce fat, and strengthen your bones.

HEALTH FLASH

Columbia. "If exercise is painful, you won't want to do it. You may even injure yourself, which will keep you from doing it at all."

That said, you still need to push yourself a bit if weight loss is your goal. You may have heard that the harder you work out, the fewer fat calories you burn. Technically, it's true—but it doesn't mean that you should cut the intensity of your exercise routine.

The math goes something like this: Suppose you were to jog three miles at a slow to moderate pace. You'd burn about 200 total calories, 60 percent of which

Make Your Workout Count

Here's a rundown of various activities, along with the approximate number of calories each burns for a 135-pound woman. Use this list to create an exercise routine that you're comfortable with.

Activity	Calories Burned (Per 30 Minutes)
Mountain biking	259
Carrying groceries upstairs	244
Swimming laps (moderate pace)	244
Running	214
Cross-country skiing (slow pace)	213
Racewalking	198
Aerobic dancing (high intensity)	183
Free-weight lifting (high intensity)	183
Stationary cycling (slow pace)	168
Playing with the kids (high intensity)	153
Calisthenics (light to moderate intensity)	137
Mowing the lawn	137
Mopping the floor	122
Walking the dog	107

would come from fat. That's 120 fat calories. If you were to run the same distance at a faster pace, you'd burn more total calories—maybe 350. Even if only 50 percent of those calories came from fat, that's still 175. You're burning more total calories and more fat calories at a higher intensity.

The upshot: To really work out for weight loss, crank up your intensity a notch or two. Even adding 5 to 10 minutes to your exercise routine each week will increase your calorie expenditure.

Incidentally, this doesn't mean you must set aside a half-hour or more each day for exercise. The latest research indicates that you can get as many benefits from 1- to 10-minute blocks of activity as from one concentrated session.

The prescription: What you burn versus what you eat is the key to weight loss. Most experts—including the American College of Sports Medicine, the Centers for Disease Control and Prevention, and the Surgeon General—agree that 30 minutes of moderate-intensity exercise at least five days a week is enough to gradually take pounds off and keep them off. "Moderate" means that you should feel slightly winded, but not exhausted, at the end of your workout. Aim to burn 150 to 200 calories a day. (To find out which activities burn the most calories, see "Make Your Workout Count.")

If You Want to Stay Slim . . .

Once you shed those extra pounds, exercise "lite"—as moderate exercise combined with active everyday tasks has been dubbed—can help you maintain a healthy weight. One study found that moderate exercisers who built physical activities such as climbing stairs and walking into their days burned as many calories (159 per day, on average), gained as much muscle, and lost as much fat as gym-goers did.

The prescription: Walking is commonly cited as the best form of moderate exercise. But climbing stairs, gardening, and carrying groceries all count toward your daily total as long as they keep you moving.

If You Want to Get Stronger . . .

In their quest to be thin, many women overlook the importance of resistance training. But consider the benefits of adding resistance training to your exercise program. You'll have more strength and stamina, you'll be less prone to injury—and you'll look better in a bathing suit. Plus, the more muscle you build, the more calories you'll burn, says Dr. Durstine. Why? Muscle tissue uses calories faster than fat tissue. Your body will be frying more calories even when you're resting.

The prescription: Aim for two to three 20-minute resistance-training sessions a week. That's in addition to your five or more 30-minute aerobic sessions a week. Use free weights (dumbbells or a barbell), do calisthenics (situps, pushups, leg raises, and the like), or try circuit-training machines at the gym.

If You Want to Outrun Your Kids . . .

Challenging your body with periods of vigorous exercise will build a stronger heart and lungs, which in turn will feed more oxygen to your muscles. Your muscles will then use that oxygen to convert food into energy—and you'll have more get-up-and-go to chase after Junior.

Once your body is in better aerobic condition, you'll be able to do more with less effort. Everyday tasks such as hauling laundry and vacuuming will cause barely a blip in your energy level. You'll even have enough zip left to shoot hoops or play a game of tag with the kids after dinner.

Sustained, intense activity is the key to pushing yourself to an aerobically fit, high-energy level, says Dr. Rippe. So try racewalking, running, aerobic dancing, cycling, rowing, cross-country skiing, or stairclimbing. You can also do interval training—alternating two to three minutes of high-intensity activity with an equal period of low-intensity activity. For instance, setting your treadmill for a long hill followed by flat terrain may get you into shape faster than steady-speed walking.

The prescription: Exercise for 20 to 60 minutes, three to five times a week, at an intensity that raises your heart rate to 70 to 85 percent of maximum. To determine your maximum heart rate, subtract your age from 220. Multiply that number by 0.70 and 0.85, and you have your maximum heart rate range.

If You Want to Improve Your Mood . . .

When you're feeling down, probably the last thing you want to do is exercise. But researchers have found that even a brisk 10-minute walk can immediately improve your state of mind. Regular exercise can give you a heightened sense of well-being.

The best news is that exercise doesn't have to be vigorous to lift your spirits. It simply needs to be continuous and rhythmic. Walking, swimming, and biking are all good options. Be sure to avoid engaging in activities that spark a competitive urge, cautions Thomas G. Plante, Ph.D., associate professor of psychology at Santa Clara University in California. Putting pressure on yourself to achieve a certain time in a 10-K run, for example, can actually make you feel worse instead of better. Besides, it doesn't get you into that distracted, meditative, "timeout" zone that's most beneficial for your mood, says Dr. Plante.

The prescription: Follow the standard recommendation for 30 minutes of moderate exercise at least five days a week. This level of activity appears to be as beneficial for the mind as for the body.

If You Want to Live Longer . . .

Pretty much any form of regular exercise can slow the aging process. Recent studies from the Cooper Aerobics Research Institute in Dallas found that moderate exercise offers many of the same health benefits as traditional, structured, gym-based programs. It reduces deaths from heart attack, stroke, cancer, and diabetes by 55 percent and extends life by up to 2½ years.

Not surprisingly, the Cooper Aerobics Research Institute and other research facilities have also found that the higher you go on the fitness scale, the longer you'll live and the healthier you'll be. By achieving a high level of aerobic fitness, you'll reduce your risk of death from the conditions mentioned above by 65 percent and possibly extend your life by three years.

The prescription: Participate in regular exercise, whether it's "lite" or high intensity. It will improve your quality of life as you get older, keeping you mobile and mentally sharp.

18

No-Sweat Ways to Burn Calories All Day

You meant to wake up early and hit the stationary bike, but the baby cried all night. You thought that you would spend your lunch break at the gym, but then the boss "delegated" another last-minute disaster. Go for a walk after dinner? Yeah, that would work—if only you didn't have to balance your checkbook.

Does this sound like your life? You're not alone.

The Surgeon General's Report on Physical Activity and Health recommends that you get 30 minutes of moderate-intensity physical activity every day. But in reality, a hectic lifestyle dominated by obligations to family, friends, and career can make carving out a half-hour for a workout seem nearly impossible.

The good news is, you have an alternative. The latest research indicates that three 10-minute sessions of activity may produce nearly the same fitness payoffs as a solid 30 minutes spent sweating it out at the gym. You can spare 10 minutes three times a day, can't you?

Here's a list of expert-recommended exercise options that can be squeezed into even the busiest schedule. Most take less than 10 minutes. Find several that appeal to you, then mix and match them so that they add up to 30 minutes of physical activity a day. In this way, you can make fitness an extension of your lifestyle—and prevent it from becoming a chore.

Programmed to Pack On Pounds

Does watching television make you fat? Not exactly. But new research has shown that people who spend more time in front of the boob tube are more sedentary, eat more snacks, and generally are more obese.

"When you're watching TV, not only do you tend to remain sedentary but you're also exposed to food commercials that might influence you to eat even more," says Steven Gortmaker, Ph.D., senior lecturer at Harvard School of Public Health.

What can you do to escape a TV-watching rut? Dr. Gortmaker offers these suggestions.

❖ Tape a piece of paper to the back of your remote control or *TV Guide*. Then every time you watch a show, write down how long you sat there and what you ate. After a week, look over your notes. "That's usually a wake-up call for people," says Dr. Gortmaker.

❖ If there's a TV in your bedroom, move it elsewhere. "Having a TV in your bedroom greatly increases your viewing time," notes Dr. Gortmaker. The less accessible the TV is, the less likely you are to vegetate in front of it.

❖ Replace at least a portion of your TV time with another activity. Start small: When you feel the urge to settle in front of the set, take a walk around the block instead. "The most important thing is that you make a conscious decision to change your habits," says Dr. Gortmaker.

HEALTH FLASH

At-Home Toners

Fitness begins at home. You have lots of opportunities to engage in a little calorie-burning activity throughout the day. Here are some examples.

1. Heating your dinner? Do knee bends as you microwave. (Be sure to stand away from the oven, though.)
2. Vacuuming? Do lunges as you push the vacuum cleaner. For proper form, keep the knee of your forward leg aligned with the heel.
3. Do biceps curls while talking on the phone. You can use a book as a makeshift dumbbell.

Work Out by the Numbers

One size seldom fits all, especially in terms of burning calories. The number of calories used up when you exercise depends on your weight. That's why charts listing the calorie-burning power of various activities usually say that the numbers are based on a certain weight. Unfortunately, the weight may not match your own.

With a calculator and some simple math, however, you can customize these charts to your weight. Just use this formula: the number of calories listed in the chart ÷ the weight used for the chart × your weight = the number of calories you'll burn.

As an example, suppose a particular chart says that a 130-pound woman can burn 384 calories per hour while horseback riding. You weigh 147 pounds. Just do the math: 384 calories ÷ 130 pounds × 147 pounds = 434 calories. In other words, you'll use up 434 calories per hour.

4. If your laundry room is in the basement, climb the stairs for a good workout.
5. Waiting for the water in the tea kettle to boil? Do half-squats, balancing yourself by placing your fingertips on the kitchen counter.
6. Rake leaves and bag them.
7. Instead of hitting the snooze alarm in the morning, do 10 minutes of stretching exercises.
8. Walk your dog. If you don't have one, volunteer to walk your neighbor's.
9. Do pushups or crunches while you watch television.
10. Wash and wax your car. Alternate hands as you go.
11. While sitting to read a book or the newspaper, tighten and release your stomach muscles.
12. Turn on the radio and dance.
13. Get a cordless phone and pace around the room as you talk.

On-the-Job Training

Your workday is so packed that you seldom have time to eat lunch, much less exercise. Never fear: With a little creativity, you can turn your workplace into a veritable gym.

14. Take the stairs to your office or to another department instead of using the elevator.
15. While sitting at your desk, grab one knee and raise it toward your chest. Lower that knee, then raise the other knee. Alternate 10 times.
16. Instead of a coffee break, opt for a fresh-air break and take a brisk walk around the block.

17. Walk to a co-worker's office to talk to her instead of using the phone.
18. Mix business with fitness. Discuss a project with a colleague as both of you take a walk.
19. Do alternate leg raises while sitting in front of your computer. Keep your abs tight.
20. Stand up, hold on to the back of your chair, and do toe raises.
21. Stand up and stretch as often as you can.
22. Extend your arms out to the sides at shoulder level and make small circles. Then make larger ones.
23. Pick up a paperweight and do biceps curls while seated at your desk.
24. Shrug your shoulders up and down to release tension.
25. Slowly and gently roll your neck from side to side.
26. Take a deep-breathing break to rejuvenate yourself. Slowly inhale and exhale.

Running around Town

If you're on the go, you're burning calories. Here are some ways to get the most out of errands and other outings.

27. Tighten your abdomen or buttocks, then release. You can do this anytime, anywhere, without anyone knowing.
28. Walk briskly everywhere—to the post office, the bank, the dry cleaner. Pump your arms.
29. While waiting in line, clench your fists at waist level and arch your shoulders back. This tones the muscles in your arms and back.
30. Take your bike to do errands.

Taking to the Road

Sitting in your car? Take advantage of your time behind the wheel by sneaking in a few energizing moves.

31. Each time you stop at a traffic light, do stretches to loosen up your neck, shoulders, and back.
32. Park your car farther from your destination and walk the rest of the way.
33. When driving a long distance, stop at a safe location every hour or so. Get out of your car and walk around, bend, and stretch. Then be on your way.

Sky-High Exercise

Whether you're traveling for business or pleasure, you don't have to leave your workout behind. You can find activities that are appropriate just about anywhere—even in an airplane, as the following tips illustrate. For more comfort and room to move, request an exit row or bulkhead seat.

34. While seated, flex your ankles to work your calf muscles.
35. Stand in the aisle and stretch your quadriceps by alternately grabbing each ankle and pulling your heel up toward your buttocks. Hold for a count of eight.
36. As you wait to use the lavatory, stretch your hamstrings by reaching toward your toes.
37. Reach up toward the ceiling, alternating your right and left hands. Do 8 to 10 times with each arm.
38. Use your arms to lift yourself from your seat.
39. Practice your travel fitness routine at home. This way, you'll know what to do when you're on the road.

Accommodating Your Workout

Hotels often have weight rooms, cardiovascular equipment, and pools for fitness-conscious clientele. Because services and facilities vary widely, call ahead to check out your fitness options.

40. Pack a couple of exercise bands for a good resistance workout. *Ione It Up*, a video by Kari Anderson, will show you how to use them. (You can order the tape from Collage Video. The company's 800 number is available by calling toll-free directory assistance.)
41. Travel with your favorite exercise video. Hotels with conference or meeting facilities often have VCRs for guest use. Request one for your room.
42. If your hotel has in-room movies, request an exercise video just as you would any other type of movie.
43. Pack a jump rope in your suitcase. Jump on a carpet or another shock-absorbing surface.
44. Call the concierge and have an exercise bike delivered to your room.
45. Go for a swim.
46. Do calisthenics such as pushups and jumping jacks in your room.
47. Walk to nearby destinations. Grab your camera and do a little sight-seeing.
48. Have the hotel's courtesy car take you to a nearby mall, so you can mall-walk.
49. Do yoga or tai chi in your room.
50. Need a personal trainer for the day? A safe walking or jogging route? Ask the hotel concierge.
51. Check whether your health club has reciprocal arrangements with a health club in the city where you're staying.

Real Options for Busy Moms

You don't have to postpone exercising until your baby or young child is older. Running around with kids can be a workout in itself. Just use a little ingenuity and put safety first.

52. Lying on your back with your knees bent, position and hold your baby on your abdomen. Raise your head and shoulders toward your baby to exercise your abs.
53. Do the "baby press": Lie on your back with your knees bent. Hold your tot firmly under the arms and place him on your chest. Lift your baby toward the ceiling as if you were doing a bench press. *Note:* Your baby must be able to hold up his head. Don't do this right after feeding.
54. While your baby crawls around, get on your hands and knees and do a few pushups.
55. Do seated calf raises with your child sitting just above your knees.
56. Work your shoulders and upper arms by lifting your baby up over your head.
57. Walk, run, or inline skate as you push the stroller. You can buy a stroller specially designed for this purpose.
58. Pull your child in a wagon.
59. Jump rope with your child.
60. While supervising your child in the swimming pool, climb in yourself and do water aerobics. Don't want to mess your hair? Do jumping jacks poolside.
61. Find fitness activities that the whole family can enjoy, like ice-skating, bike riding, or hiking, and make them a part of your weekly schedule.
62. Enjoy a "walk and roll" with your kids—walk while they ride their bikes or skate.
63. After dropping off your child at soccer practice, take a walk around the playing field.
64. Join a health club that provides on-site babysitting services.
65. Visit a bike shop and check out the parent-child tandem bikes.
66. Round up your kids for an informal dance contest. Put on a CD and have fun together making up new steps.
67. Make a fitness appointment with yourself—and keep it. Write it in your appointment book in ink.
68. Exchange babysitting services with a friend twice a week, so each of you can work out at the gym.

Walk Off Extra Pounds

Walking is the world's most accommodating exercise.

While you walk, you can do all manner of other things. Henry David Thoreau thought lofty thoughts while strolling around Walden Pond. Walking to his day job at the Hartford Accident and Indemnity Company, Wallace Stevens composed Pulitzer Prize–winning poetry.

Not in the mood for poetry or philosophizing? Take a friend along on your walk, and the two of you can just catch up while you stroll. Or take your dry cleaning and stop off at the Quik Clean on your amble.

Walking is simplicity itself. There's no need to count repetitions or keep score while you walk. And there's no need to tote around special equipment or search out special environs. You can walk virtually anywhere.

"There's no reason a person can't engage in a walking program on a regular basis," says John Duncan, Ph.D., professor of clinical research at Texas Woman's University in Denton and author of several studies on walking.

Better Health, Step by Step

Walking offers a multitude of health benefits. A regular walking program will help you lose weight and keep it off. It'll help control diabetes. One study

Skip TV Exercise Machines

Channel-surf through the sea of infomercials aired on Saturday morning TV, and you quickly realize two things. One, cartoons aren't that bad. And two, you need to get a hobby. Yet this hokey testimonial television makes a lot of money selling stuff, including exercise equipment.

The American Council on Exercise (ACE), a non-profit health and fitness organization, commissioned a group of exercise scientists to check out the claims of three types of exercise gear sold on television. The result: All received low marks.

Air gliders, which move your legs and arms as you stride on suspended foot platforms, had questionable stability, durability, and adjustability. Even when people put out maximum effort on these popular devices, the workout tended to be less effective than a quick walk or a slow jog. Most air gliders cost about $200.

Aerobic riders are pedal/push-pull machines that can cost up to $600. The researchers found that a person burned approximately 25 percent fewer calories on an aerobic rider than during a similar workout on a treadmill.

And none of the $75-plus abdominal trainers—curved bars that claim to tighten tummies—was more effective than doing simple, unaided stomach crunches.

According to Richard Cotton, an exercise physiologist and ACE spokesperson, TV exercise machines aren't all bad. "If they help get someone started, fine," he says. "But when the equipment doesn't meet expectations, it leads to disappointment and discouragement."

If you are itching to spend money on exercise, Cotton recommends joining a health club or hiring a personal trainer. At the very least, wait until the equipment you want reaches the retail market, where its price drops dramatically.

HEALTH FLASH

found that women who spend just three hours a week walking at a moderate three-mile-per-hour pace are less likely to have heart attacks or strokes. Walking makes your heart work harder, so it grows stronger. And walking lowers your blood pressure while boosting levels of HDL cholesterol (the good kind) in your bloodstream.

Walking builds other muscles besides the heart. Stronger muscles do a better job keeping joints in proper alignment, thereby reducing the wear and tear that contributes to osteoarthritis. And some studies suggest that walking can keep your bones strong, helping you outpace osteoporosis.

As if all those benefits weren't enough, here's the cream on top. Research has shown that a regular constitutional boosts mental health, easing depression and anxiety. "Walking is one of nature's tranquilizers," Dr. Duncan says. "It reduces the production of stress hormones, helping you calm down and put life in perspective."

The faster you walk, the greater the benefits. For instance, you'll burn calories and build muscle quicker. "When you're walking five miles an hour, you're getting the same fitness benefits you would if you were jogging—with a significantly lower risk of injury," Dr. Duncan says. "The injury rate for walking is far lower than for virtually any other activity."

Unlike jogging, which has you jostling up and down like a pogo stick, walking is a low-impact affair. When you walk, one of your feet is always on the ground. No bouncing. No pounding. So walking is kind to your joints and vertebrae.

It's a particularly good exercise choice if you have arthritis or if you're overweight (since extra pounds also put extra stress on your joints). "And walking is an ideal exercise option if you have lower-back pain. It'll strengthen your back muscles without giving your disks a drubbing," says exercise physiologist Carol Espel, a contributor to *The YMCA Walk Reebok Instructor Manual* and general manager of Equinox of New York City, a health and fitness club in Westchester, New York.

Select the Right Shoes

To start walking, all you need are a good pair of shoes and some pointers on posture and pace. Sore shins, one of the very few hazards of walking, often result from the wrong footwear, Espel says. So keep these thoughts in mind when selecting your shoes.

Shop late. Your feet swell a bit over the course of the day. So a pair of shoes that fits at 9:00 in the morning may pinch a bit by dusk. Shop in the afternoon or at night, when your feet tend to be largest.

Pay the freight. Yes, lots of athletic shoes are very expensive. And you don't need the nuclear-powered pair that breaks the $100 mark. But you should buy high-quality walking shoes. To do so, you may have to spend between $50 and $75.

When you're shoe-shopping, Espel suggests looking for a pair with the following features.

❖ A heel that slopes up in back. A beveled heel makes rolling your foot from heel to toe easy. This is the proper stepping technique and will help you avoid straining your shins. Nothing insults a sensitive shin like slapping your whole foot flat down on the ground.

❖ A flexible forefoot. A rolling heel-toe gait also requires a flexible sole. Look for a shoe with a sole that bends easily.

❖ Cushioning under the heel and forefoot. Even though walking is low impact, your foot still needs some shock absorption.

❖ A spacious toebox. Each time you roll onto your toes, those little digits move forward and far outward. Give them sufficient space, in a shoe with a capacious toe.

Proper Pedestrian Posture

To get the maximum benefit from walking, you need proper walking posture, Espel says. Here are two things to keep in mind.

Keep your chin up. When walking, you should hold your head high and look toward the horizon, not down at your feet. "Looking at your feet pulls your upper body down and can cause lower-back pain," Espel explains. Your head should be in line with your spine. And your shoulders should be back, so your rib cage is lifted and opened up.

Involve your arms. Your arms should swing as you walk. If they don't, you won't get the upper-body benefit of walking. But beware of flailing your arms. Let them swing freely but not excessively. Keeping your elbows close to your sides as they swing should help you find the right arm rhythm and movement.

Learn to Step Lively

According to an ancient Chinese adage, "A journey of a thousand miles must begin with a single step." Here are some tips for your first few steps to lifetime fitness.

Start slowly. Spend the first five minutes of each walk just ambling along at your normal walking pace, Espel advises. No strain, no huffing or puffing. This gives your muscles an opportunity to warm up before you make demands on them. That's important, because cold muscles are more vulnerable to exercise-related injuries.

Do some stretches. Here are a few simple pre-walk exercises.

❖ Stretch your hips. While standing with your feet shoulder-width apart, step your right foot forward about 12 inches. Tuck your buttocks under your hips, and pull in your stomach muscles. When you do, you should feel a stretch at the front of your upper left hip and your upper left thigh. Hold for 15 seconds, then repeat on the other side. You may want to hold onto a table or something else sturdy for support.

❖ Save your shins. While standing, cross your left calf and foot over your right shin and foot. Then bend your left knee, pointing your left foot so that only the toe of your left shoe touches the ground. (Think ballerina.) Then press your right shin into your left calf. You should feel a mild stretch in your left shin. Hold for 15 seconds, then repeat the move—this time, crossing your right calf and foot over your left shin and foot. Again, you may want to hold onto something sturdy for balance.

Pick up the pace. Once you've stretched, you're ready to walk again. The important thing when you're starting out is to choose a comfortable pace. Don't worry if you're not moving as fast as everyone else. You'll pick up speed in due time. "You don't need to huff and puff at first," Espel says. "Walking should be enjoyable, not stressful or painful."

Go around the block. If the last long walk you took was down the aisle of the Hillcrest High auditorium during graduation, start short. Walk around the block or, if you're in the country, past four telephone poles. You want a distance that will take you about 10 minutes to cover, Espel says. Do it three times a week. Remember: Walk at a comfortable pace.

Walk farther. When walking for 10 minutes or so three times a week is no longer a challenge, add distance. Make it 12 to 15 minutes a pop, Espel says. Gradually work up to 30 minutes three times weekly. Then aim for 30 minutes five times weekly. If you want to lose weight, Dr. Duncan suggests walking for 40 to 60 minutes four or five times a week.

Walk faster. Over time, you'll find that you can also pick up your pace and still feel comfortable. A good rule of thumb: Walk fast enough that you can talk but you can't sing. To get all of the cardiovascular benefits that walking offers, you must walk at a pace of at least three miles an hour—about strolling pace—or faster, says Dr. Duncan. So make that your minimum goal.

Shorten your stride. Continue to pick up the pace, and your benefits are compounded, Dr. Duncan says. Paradoxically, the secret to walking faster is taking smaller steps. "Most people think that to move faster, they should take longer strides," Espel notes. "But quicker, shorter steps make you move faster." That's because your hips can rotate faster when you shorten your stride. And if you pump your arms faster, your feet have to follow.

Cool your heels. Cool down by spending the last five minutes of your walk strolling, Espel says. Then finish up with some basic stretches, so you don't get all stiff and rigid. You can repeat the stretches you did after your warmup. You can also try the following ones.

❖ Roll your feet. This gives your hardworking shins and calves a good after-walk stretch. Stand with your feet 6 to 12 inches apart, slowly roll up onto your toes, and hold this position for a count of two. Then roll onto the outsides of your feet and hold for two. Next, roll back onto your heels and lift your toes. Hold for a count of two. Finish with your feet flat on the ground. Repeat up to

10 times. You may want to hold onto something sturdy for balance. "You need to be careful when rolling your feet and ankles," Espel says.

❖ Relax your back. Lying on your back with your knees pulled toward your chest, place your left hand on the outside of your left thigh (about mid-thigh) and your right hand on the outside of your right thigh. Then use your hands to pull your knees toward your chest. Hold for 15 seconds.

❖ Stretch your hamstrings. Lying on your back, bend your left knee so that your foot is flat on the floor. Extend your right leg straight up toward the ceiling. Remember to keep your back and hips down on the floor. Hold the stretch for 15 to 30 seconds, then switch legs.

For a Change of Pace . . .

Once you're comfortable with a basic walking routine, you can add variety and challenge with specialized workouts. Here are a few examples.

Experience ups and downs. Hill walking is just what it sounds like—walking up and down hills. Repeatedly. This gives your heart a more strenuous workout. It can also help tone your tush, Espel says. To try hill walking, find some moderately steep hills and tread up and down them for 20 minutes.

Add intervals. Walk as fast as you can for 30 seconds, then slow down to your usual pace for 90 seconds. Keep repeating the pattern: 30 seconds fast, 90 seconds slow. That's interval walking. It burns more calories and gives your stamina a bigger boost than "regular" walking. Aim for seven fast-slow cycles in a row, Espel says.

Go the distance. Covering more than four miles at a time qualifies as distance walking. "This is something you can do when you're preparing for an event like a 5-K walking race," Espel explains. Racing adds a competitive element to walking—an extra incentive for Type A folks. To find out about races in your area (most running races welcome walkers), contact your local sporting goods store or YMCA.

Vary Your Vistas

Since you can walk virtually anywhere, why limit yourself to the same old stretch of sidewalk? Explore the following new frontiers.

Walk with the animals. Take a walking tour of a zoo. Or if you prefer flora to fauna, visit a botanical garden.

Make the rounds downtown. Most cities—even small ones—are home to enough attractions to warrant a self-guided tour or two. Call the chamber of commerce in your town (or one nearby) and ask for a map. Then check out the local sights.

Extra Steps Really Do Count

Walking is a great way to whittle away pounds and inches. So anything that you can do to add a few steps to your daily routine will benefit your shape and your dress size. Here are some suggestions.

❖ Take a lap around the supermarket or the mall before you start shopping. (This is a great way to look for sales.)

❖ Store nonperishables such as canned food, paper products, and cleansers in the basement. Then when you need something, you get to make a quick trip up and down the stairs. No basement? Store the items in the attic instead.

❖ Get your wastebasket out from under your desk. Put it in a far corner of your office, or better yet, use one down the hall. Just don't save all your trash for one trip.

❖ Soccer (or any other sit-on-the-bleachers-sports) moms: Get off the bench. Walk around the field during the game. Chances are you'll get a better view. (And in cold weather, you'll stay warm, too.)

Head into the woods. Odds are you live within driving distance of a hiking trail or two. Most state maps show local, state, and national parks, and many of those parks have hiking paths. Stores that sell outdoor sporting goods are sure to have local walking books or detailed trail guides. Or call your state parks department (the number is listed in the Blue Pages) to request free maps of trails near home.

Hike Hawaii. Imagine yourself traversing the black sand of Kings Highway Coastal Trail in Maui, through lush tropical vegetation to ancient village ruins. Then do it. Country Walkers and Cross Country International—just two of a number of organizations that offer walking tours through the world's most scenic landscapes—will get you there.

Walking tour outfits like Country Walkers lead organized hikes both in the United States and abroad. Cross Country International specializes in walking and hiking tours of the British Isles. The organizations usually arrange for accommodations and meals, so all you have to do is put one foot in front of the other. You can contact Country Walkers at P. O. Box 180, Waterbury, VT 05676, or Cross Country International at P. O. Box 1170, Millbrook, NY 12545. Ask your travel agent for information about other walking tours.

20

Slim Down and Shape Up in 30 Days

O ne month until your dream vacation. Or your class reunion. Or your niece's wedding. Whatever the occasion, you wanted to take off a few pounds so you'd look your svelte, sensational best. Now you've run out of time.

Well, don't pack in your plans just yet. With a little commitment—no more than one hour a day for the next 30 days—you can have the shape you want. Yes, you'll have to sweat a bit. But a month from now, you'll agree that the pay-off is worth it. In fact, you'll look and feel so good that you may decide to continue your new fitness routine for the long run.

The following workout—developed with assistance from exercise physiologist Liz Neporent, author of *Weight Training for Dummies*—can easily be done at home. It requires just a few pieces of equipment: a floor mat or thick carpeting, a chair, and a set of dumbbells (3 to 5 pounds if you're a beginner, 5 to 8 pounds if you're basically in good shape).

You'll notice that the workout is divided into three segments: lower body, upper body, and abdominals. No one segment is repeated on consecutive days. This allows your various muscle groups to rest and recover between sessions. When doing the maximum number of repetitions per exercise becomes easy, you can increase the intensity of your workout by lifting more weight or slowing the movements. (Have you ever tried doing a superslow pushup? If so, you know how hard it is.)

Remember to warm up before your workout—try 5 minutes of jumping rope or marching in place—and to cool down afterward. Also, don't forsake

Treadmill Beats Stationary Bike by a Mile

H E A L T H   F L A S H

Researchers at the Medical College of Wisconsin and Veterans Affairs Medical Center in Milwaukee recently tested six indoor exercise machines—a treadmill, a stairclimbing machine, a rowing machine, a cross-country ski machine, and two stationary bikes (one with movable handlebars, the other without). Their goal was to find out which contraption coaxes the biggest calorie burn at certain rates of perceived exertion.

Their winner? The treadmill.

In fact, when the study's participants exercised what they described as "somewhat hard," they burned 40 percent more calories by running on the treadmill than by pedaling on the stationary bikes.

Second- and third-place calorie-burning kudos went to the stairclimbing machine and the rowing machine, respectively.

aerobic exercise. It's an indispensable component of your shape-up program. Aim for 30 minutes of aerobic activity—such as brisk walking, running, cycling, or swimming—every day.

Note: If you're out of shape, check with your doctor before beginning any exercise program.

Lower Body

Switch between the upper-body and lower-body sequences, so you're including them in your workout on alternate days. For each of the following exercises, do one set of 8 to 15 repetitions.

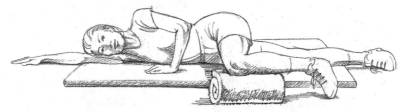

Inner-Thigh Lift

Lie on your right side with a rolled–up towel beneath your lower left leg and your head on your right arm, as shown. Place your left hand on the floor in front of you, palm down, for balance. Bend your left leg and rest your left knee on the towel in front of you at hip level. Raise your right leg about six to eight inches off the floor, then lower. Do all of your repetitions before switching sides.

Squat

Stand with your feet a little more than hip-width apart. Slowly lower your torso until your calves and thighs form a 90-degree angle. Keep your back straight, look forward, and don't let your knees go past your toes. Slowly return to the starting position.

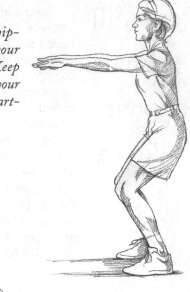

Quad Tightener

Sit on the floor with your back against a wall and both legs extended in front of you. Bend your left leg and hug it to your body. Place a rolled-up towel directly under your right knee, then gently press down your right knee while flexing your quads (in your upper thigh). Your heel will lift off the floor slightly. Squeeze and hold for five seconds, then return to the starting position. Do all of your repetitions before switching legs.

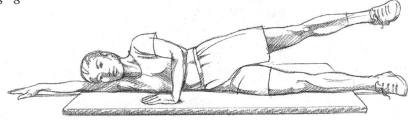

Outer-Thigh Lift

Lie on your right side with your head on your right arm, as shown. Place your left hand on the floor in front of you, palm down, for balance. Keeping your right leg straight, slowly raise your left leg about 8 to 12 inches off the floor, then lower it. Do all of your repetitions before switching sides.

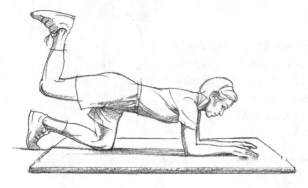

Kneeling Hamstring Curl

Position yourself on your hands and knees. Your elbows should be directly below your shoulders, and your knees should be below your hips. Your hands should be palms down. Keeping your right knee bent, raise your leg until your right thigh is parallel to the floor. Extend your right leg straight out behind you, then bend it again. Do all of your repetitions before switching legs.

Upper Body

The following exercises strengthen and tone the muscles of your shoulders, chest, back, and upper arms. For each exercise, do one set of 8 to 15 repetitions. Include the upper-body sequence in your workout every other day.

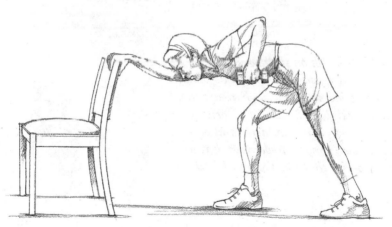

One-Arm Row

Stand a few feet behind the back of a chair with your legs shoulder-width apart and your right leg slightly in front of your left. Holding a dumbbell in your left hand, bend at the waist to place your right hand on the chair back. Make sure that your head, neck, and back are in line. Let your left arm drop down, then slowly bend your elbow until the dumbbell is at chest level. Keep your elbow pointing behind you and your left arm close to your body. Return to the starting position. Do all of your repetitions before switching arms.

Shoulder Press

Stand with your feet shoulder-width apart and hold a dumbbell in each hand. Raise the dumbbells so that your elbows are level with your shoulders and your palms are facing forward. Breathe in, then exhale while stretching your arms up in the air. Slowly return the dumbbells to your shoulders.

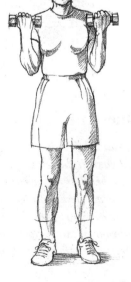

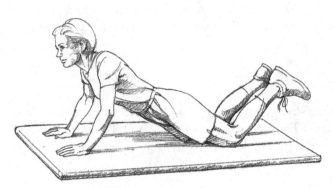

Pushup

Place your hands on the floor about shoulder-width apart, with your palms down and your fingers facing forward. Either extend your legs straight behind you or bend your knees. Keeping your head, neck, and back in line, bend your elbows to lower your body until it almost touches the floor. Then push back up.

Biceps Curl

Stand with your feet shoulder-width apart and hold a dumbbell in each hand. Let your arms drop down to your sides, with your palms facing in. Slowly bend your elbows and raise the dumbbells to your shoulders. Your palms should still be facing in. Hold, then return to the starting position.

Triceps Kickback

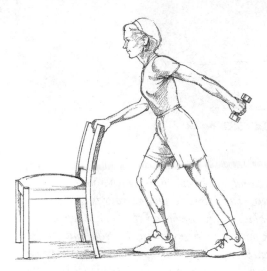

Stand a few feet behind the back of a chair with your legs shoulder-width apart and your right leg slightly in front of your left. Holding a dumbbell in your left hand, bend over slightly to place your right hand on the chair back. Make sure that your head, neck, and back are in line. Bend your left arm and hold the dumbbell at chest level. Then slowly extend your left arm behind you as shown, being careful not to lock your elbow. Do all of your repetitions before switching arms.

Abdominals

On days when you include abdominal exercises in your workout, do them first. If you wait until the end of your workout, you may be too tired to bother. For each exercise, do three or four sets of 8 to 15 repetitions. Rest for 30 to 90 seconds between sets. The entire sequence should take approximately 10 minutes. Repeat two or three times per week, preferably not on consecutive days.

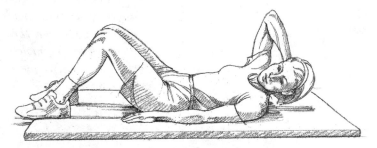

Oblique Twist

Lie on the floor with your back flat and your knees bent, hip-width apart. Fold your right arm behind your head and place your left arm on the floor, palm down. Raise your right shoulder, aiming toward your left knee. Don't try to touch your elbow to your knee. Return to the starting position. Do all of your repetitions before switching arms.

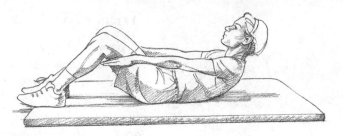

Crunch

Lie on the floor with your back flat and knees bent, hip-width apart. Place your hands straight out in front of you, with your palms down and your fingers pointing toward your feet. Lift your shoulder blades a few inches off the floor. Keep your eyes on the ceiling; do not crane your neck forward when you lift. Instead, imagine that you are trying to touch the ceiling with your chest. Remain in this position while contracting and releasing your abdominal muscle 8 to 12 times. Don't let your upper back touch the floor. Then return to the starting position.

Air Bicycle

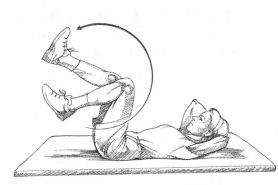

Lie on the floor with your back flat and your knees bent, hip-width apart. Place your hands behind your head, which should be raised slightly off the floor. Keeping your knees bent, lift them in the air so that your legs and torso form a 90-degree angle (your back should be flat against the floor throughout). Make 10 to 15 complete rotations with your legs, as if you were riding a bicycle.

Excuse-Proof Weight Loss

21

I'll start tomorrow." Those three infamous words mark the beginning of the end for any weight-loss program. They precede all the no-nos, like reaching for a honey-dipped chocolate doughnut. Or skipping step-acrobics class. Or trading your morning walk for some more Zzzs. But it's the reasons behind those three words that are really to blame. The excuses for why you can't, won't, shouldn't have to change your life (at least not until tomorrow).

Old habits really do die hard, and new routines don't just spring to life. You have to be convinced that a healthier lifestyle is preferable to your current one. Not being altogether sold on the benefits of such a switch is what excuses are often about. But you can overcome your own avoidance tactics. The key is to have counterexcuses to help you tackle (and reverse) every objection you can come up with. With that in mind, here are eight common excuses for not starting or sticking with a weight-loss plan—and 18 great ways to bid them adieu.

"Just Thinking about Losing Weight Makes Me Feel Deprived"

If you want to slim down, you have to make some lifestyle changes. They go with the territory. But rather than dwelling on what you can't eat or can't do, focus on your options and opportunities. Here's how.

Add, don't subtract. Aim to improve upon your favorite things. If you're into watching television, for example, that's fine. But buy a stationary bicycle and pedal while you're glued to the tube, suggests Pat Manocchia, a personal trainer and owner of LaPalestra Center for Preventive Medicine in New York City. "Add things to your life so you don't feel like you're missing something," he says.

Same goes for food. If eating out with friends is a special pleasure, go right ahead—but make some adjustments, says Ellie Krieger, R.D., a nutritionist in private practice in New York City. Split an entrée with a friend and order a big salad to complement it. Or eat half your entrée and take home the rest.

Focus on the perks. There's no greater motivator than thinking of how good you'll feel and how healthy you'll be when you lose weight. "When you're fit, you participate more in life," Manocchia says. "You can get out on the slopes and ski with your family instead of waiting for them back at the lodge. You can play ball with your kids." Also, when you go shopping, you'll have an easier time finding clothes that fit.

"I Can't Stay Motivated"

Maybe you've tried to slim down in the past. But two or three weeks into your program, you found yourself slipping back into old habits—like parking yourself in front of the TV after dinner instead of going for a walk. You could have been changing too much too soon. This time around, follow this advice.

Set reasonable goals. Many people sabotage themselves by expecting too

Restart without Soreness

Everyone misses a workout or two now and then. Vacations, work deadlines, winter weather, even boredom can derail the most committed exercisers. The worst part is getting started again. That first walk, run, or aerobics class after a layoff can leave you aching. The trick is to ease back into it.

As a general rule, the amount of time you missed exercising should equal the amount of time you give yourself to return to your previous level. Say you were cycling 15 miles in an hour before you went to Florida for two weeks. Your first week back, do 10 miles in an hour. At the beginning of the next week, take up to 1½ hours to ride 15 miles. Then gradually increase your speed each day until you're back to your routine by the start of the third week.

much. If you're trying to lose weight, Krieger says, aim for no more than a pound or two a week. If you push for more, the pounds might not stay off. Or you might get discouraged and backslide.

Similarly, set exercise goals that are neither too easy nor too hard. "A successful program is slightly challenging but attainable," notes Manocchia. If you are able to walk for just 10 minutes a day this week, congratulate yourself—then up your goal to 15 minutes a day next week, and 20 minutes a day the week after that. But don't push yourself by jumping straight into an hour of walking. You'll only set yourself up for disappointment.

Think small. "You can change your whole life a few little things at a time," Krieger says. So plan three small changes that you can make right now. For instance, snack on fruit instead of potato chips, or eat more salad and less meat. When these have become everyday habits, move on to more small changes. In time, these little switcheroos will add up to weight loss.

Work out with a buddy. Take your walks with a friend or hit the gym with a family member. This makes you accountable to them and much less likely to blow off your workout. Choose someone at a similar level of fitness so that the two of you are pretty much in sync and can share the satisfaction of each other's progress.

"Making Low-Fat Versions of My Favorite Recipes Is Hard"

Low-fat cooking has long had a reputation as a time-consuming, costly affair requiring special equipment and ingredients. It doesn't have to be that way, if you go about it right. These tips can help.

Cut half the fat. Halving the fat in many recipes is a breeze—and you probably won't even notice a difference. Krieger substitutes kidney beans for half the beef in her family's traditionally meaty chili, and it still tastes hearty and delicious. Other easy cuts: Replace half the cheese in lasagna with spinach. Or use half the butter when you whip up mashed potatoes.

Just add vegetables. Cooking with more veggies and less meat, cheese, and other higher-fat foods is one of the easiest ways to eat low-fat without making drastic changes in your family's favorite recipes. Or you can vary your part of the family's meal. For instance, if everyone else is eating mashed potatoes, bake a potato for yourself and enjoy it with a little salt, pepper, and fresh chives.

Make the obvious substitutions. Use skim milk and nonfat cheese instead of the whole-fat stuff. Buy nonfat or low-fat spaghetti sauce, salad dressing, and the like. All these little changes really add up.

"Low-Fat Foods Taste Terrible"

There was a time when nonfat and low-fat foods tasted only slightly better than the cardboard they were packaged in. But they've come a long way. Even low-fat potato chips taste very much like the real thing. You're bound to find something to please your palate if you follow this advice.

Choose naturally low-fat edibles. Fresh peeled shrimp in tangy cocktail sauce. Savory grilled chicken or vegetable kabobs. A peach so ripe that the juice runs down your chin. The best part is, you don't have to hunt down the low-fat versions of mouthwatering foods like these. They're naturally, deliciously low in fat just as they are.

Keep your meals interesting. Give your mouth something to sing about by trying a new nonfat or low-fat food every week. Krieger suggests creating a basic shopping list, then adding a new item each week. Just make sure that your addition is nonfat or low-fat. Some examples: fresh papaya, a new cereal, fruit juice ice pops, or flavored coffee. Spice things up even more by having a taste-testing party with your friends.

Develop a change of taste. You weren't born to love chocolate-chip cheesecake. So be sure to give yourself a couple of weeks to adjust to low-fat foods. For instance, drink low-fat milk even if it tastes like water to start with. Before long, you'll find that a glass of the whole stuff seems as thick as paint.

"Counting Fat Grams Is Too Complicated"

The good news: Counting fat grams isn't really necessary on a day-to-day basis. You just need a general sense of which foods are high in fat and which aren't. No doubt you're already off to a good start.

Get the Energy to Change

Perhaps the most crucial step in making lifestyle changes is to realize that change does require a lot of extra energy, says Glenna Salsbury, a motivational speaker and author of *The Art of the Fresh Start: How to Make and Keep Your New Year's Resolutions for a Lifetime.* "To succeed, you have to find ways to enhance your emotional, mental, and spiritual energy supply every day," she explains. Here's how.

Get over it already. The more you worry and argue with yourself about how, say, you can't seem to lose those 20 pounds, the more depressed, anxious, and exhausted you'll become. Just deal with it. Once you simply and fully accept that you weigh more than you want to, you're relieved of tremendous stress and strain. And this can be the very trigger that injects you with fresh energy. "Suddenly, you'll find yourself able to do the very thing you were struggling with," Salsbury says.

Focus on what you want. Cultivate a clear image of your goal. See yourself at your ideal weight, physically fit and energetic, happy, and healthy. While you're at it, forget the how of getting there. "Let the how evolve and surprise you," Salsbury says. "The answers will automatically come when you're clear about where you're trying to go."

Do something different. Shake up your usual routine. Take a new route to work. In the shower, lather yourself from toe to head rather than from head to toe. Instead of your usual black coffee, stir your java with a cinnamon stick. Altering the smallest things in your everyday routine snaps you out of the almost hypnotic trance that habits create and gives you a fresh view of life.

Find something you're passionate about. Think about something you've always wanted to do—and it doesn't necessarily have to be related to your healthy lifestyle change. Then go and do it. Learn to ski. Drive coast-to-coast. Research and write your family's history. "Creating a new focus in which you're passionately interested brings life to your mind and spirit," Salsbury says. "And before you know it, the change you've been struggling with is well on its way."

Know where you stand. When you're ready to start living a low-fat lifestyle, figure out just once exactly how much fat you're eating. "Think of it as a wake-up call," Krieger says. For comparison, remember that your fat intake should not exceed 50 to 60 grams a day.

Check labels occasionally. You don't have to study food labels every time you go to the supermarket. Read them once in a while to educate yourself and make good decisions. Do you really want all that fat from one measly slice of cheese? After a while, you'll have a pretty good idea of where fat is coming from and how to avoid it without keeping a running tally throughout the day.

"I'm Too Out of Shape to Exercise"

Inactivity is no excuse to remain inactive. Of course, you should check with your doctor before launching a workout program. Once she gives you a clean bill of health, you're set to get in shape. Just remember this bit of advice.

Start slowly. Walk for 10 minutes or just 5. Lift five-pound dumbbells or just one-pounders. The point is, stick with what you're able to do, as little as that may seem to be. And measure your progress against your own goals, not anyone else's. You'll be amazed at how quickly you slim down.

"I'm Too Tired to Exercise"

You say that you can barely muster the energy to tie your shoes, let alone work out for 30 minutes. Maybe you're not fueling yourself properly. Try these timely tips.

Eat first. Have a light meal a couple hours before exercising or a snack about an hour before, Krieger advises. Otherwise, your blood sugar—your body's energy supply—will run low, and you'll poop out too quickly. As few as 100 calories (say, a piece of bread or fruit) will give you the boost you need.

Eat later. Within two hours of a workout, have a meal or at least a small snack. That's when your body is most efficient at turning food into energy and storing it so you can draw on it the next time you exercise.

"I Don't Have Time to Exercise"

If there was a popularity contest for excuses, this one would win hands down. The problem is not that you don't have time but that you have something better to do—or at least you think you do. Exercise should be treated as a priority, even if that means juggling your daily routine to accommodate it.

Mark your calendar. "The President of the United States has time to exercise," Manocchia says. "So do you." The trick is to schedule it. Pull out your calendar and write in (in pen) at least three weekly workout appointments.

Find your best time. Just because you see joggers running around your neighborhood at 7:00 A.M. doesn't mean you have to be out there, too. Figure out when you have the time and the energy to exercise: first thing in the morning before everyone else wakes up, right before lunch, after work to loosen up, or maybe a half-hour after dinner. Some people even find that their prime workout time is late at night. Whatever works for you, do it.

The Scale Won't Budge! Now What?

Y ou're still doing the same things that peeled off the first 5, 10, or 50 pounds. You've kept up your daily walk, and you're a role model for low fat eating. So why does your scale seem to be stuck on the same number?

You're on a plateau. Join the club. It happens all the time to people losing weight. "Plateaus can happen when you're doing the same things that you always were, diet- and exercise-wise," says Terri Brownlee, R.D., dietitian at the Duke University Diet and Fitness Center in Durham, North Carolina.

What has changed is you.

The smaller you are, the fewer calories you require. So the diet and exercise program that helped you get from 190 pounds down to 160 may not be burning enough calories to get you to your goal of 145.

This doesn't mean you have to swear off satisfying meals or walk to the other side of the state and back to get rid of more pounds. You just need to evaluate and adjust your weight-loss game plan. "Instead of getting down on yourself, try to understand what's not working and rethink your strategy," advises Cathy Nonas, R.D., administrative director of the Theodore B. VanItallie Center for Nutrition and Weight Management at St. Luke's–Roosevelt Hospital in New York City.

That's what Cathy Upchurch did when she hit a two-month plateau after losing 70 pounds. "I kept on giving myself pep talks and refused to give up," Upchurch recalls. "I kept telling myself that I was an athletic person underneath it all and that there were all these fun things I wanted to do." Eventually, she lost another 70 pounds—and she has kept it all off.

Thousands of women have encountered and overcome weight-loss plateaus. With the right attitude and a few new weapons in your arsenal, you, too, can win in the battle of the bulge.

Pinpoint the Problem

One of the first things you need to do is to identify what may have caused you to reach a weight-loss plateau in the first place. This means specific and careful evaluation of your eating and exercise habits. "Once you see what the problems are, you can get back on track," says Pamela Walker, Ph.D., a clinical psychologist at the Cooper Aerobics Center in Dallas. "It shifts the focus from 'something is wrong with me' to problem-solving." So ask yourself these two questions.

1. Have your portions expanded as your waistline has shrunk? "Many people who experience success start getting overconfident and complacent," notes Dr. Walker. "Portions start creeping up, and sweets start reappearing."

2. Has your exercise routine taken a backseat to less strenuous activity? Exercise is always one of the first things to go. Walks get shorter or get skipped completely.

Careful examination of eating and exercise logs can pinpoint areas where your guard may be down. Are you routinely getting your lunch from a vending machine rather than taking something healthy from home? Or skipping your evening workout to watch a couple of hours of television? "It makes you accountable to yourself," says Dr. Walker. "You may be shocked to see that you did start eating more and exercising less."

Get Calories under Control

No matter how you got on the plateau, the answer to blasting off it is to shake things up. You need to start burning more calories than you're taking in. Don't despair—it's not as hard as it sounds. These tips will help you rein in the number of calories you consume.

Measure your portions. Arm yourself with measuring devices such as a scale or measuring cups, so you don't have to rely on your eyes (or your stomach), says Nonas. Once you're familiar with what your portion sizes should be, you need only measure from time to time to make sure you're still on track. Keep portions reasonable. But don't put limits on plain veggies, raw or cooked. And aim for three to five servings of fruit a day.

Shortcut portion control. Stock up on prepackaged low-fat meals. Food labels help you keep track of your calorie and fat intakes and save you the job of measuring portions when time is tight.

Try a meal substitute. Liquid meals can be helpful, especially when you're on the run. This shouldn't become a long-term strategy, but it can help break a plateau.

Fill up on whole foods. Bananas, carrots, and air-popped popcorn pack more fiber and fewer calories than reduced-fat cakes and cookies. You'll feel full on less food.

Postpone dinner. Eating a half-hour or even an hour later than usual may be just what you need to take the edge off late-night munchies.

Drink up. "Put a liter of water on your desk and make sure you drink it by the end of the day," says Nonas. Filling up on water during the day can help make portion control easier at meals.

Limit mealtimes. So you stuck to your portion, but then you ate your kids' leftovers. Before you knew it, you were noshing ad infinitum. "It's important to do things that signal the end of the meal, such as brushing your teeth," says Nonas. Or set a timer when you sit down to dinner. When it goes off, that's your cue to get up from the table.

Go for More Burn

While the strategies above will whittle away at your calorie intake, that's only part of the equation. You must also find ways to burn more calories. Here are some suggestions.

Add a minute. "Gradually extend the length of your workouts," advises J. P. Slovak, fitness director at the Cooper Fitness Center in Dallas. A few extra minutes here and there can go a long way toward producing real results.

Lift some weights. To combat the decrease in metabolism that often comes with weight loss, increase your muscle mass. Muscles burn more calories than fat does, even when you're sleeping. And they take up less space, so you look slimmer.

Try something new. You're not the only one who gets bored on the stationary bike. Your muscles do, too. If you always work the same muscles in the same way, they become very efficient. Then they don't burn as many calories as when you first started doing the activity, explains Tedd Mitchell, M.D., medical director of the Cooper Wellness Program in Dallas. If you want to shake up your metabolism, work your muscles in new ways by cross-training. If you're walking, try swimming. If you're running, try boxing. No one activity should ever become too easy for you.

Add some intervals. Invigorate your workout with short blasts of very intense exercise. "Try not to mosey along at the same pace," says Dr. Mitchell.

"Sprint for an interval if you're running. Pedal really fast on the bike if you're cycling." Intervals make working out more exciting and challenging, and they also help burn extra calories.

Go the long way. "You don't need to have gym clothes on to get exercise," says Kyle McInnis, Ph.D., professor in the department of human performance and fitness at the University of Massachusetts in Boston. Walk to the second-floor bathroom, rather than the closest one, or do your photocopying at the machine down the hall. "Accumulating physical activity throughout the day, such as walking more and taking the stairs, adds up," he explains.

Is It a Plateau or Your Ideal Weight?

If despite your best efforts you can't seem to shed those pounds, you may not be on a plateau at all. Rather, you may have reached your ideal weight.

How can you tell the difference? If you're, say, 70 pounds more than what most weight tables recommend for your height, chances are you're on a plateau. If you're merely 10 pounds more, then it might be time to accept your weight. In between? That's a gray area.

Ideal weight varies among individuals. The term itself has become a statistical figure generated by insurance people who are telling you what to weigh to live the longest based on averages. "That's something very different," says David Levitsky, Ph.D., professor of nutrition and psychology at Cornell University in Ithaca, New York.

So if you're in that gray area, here are some things to consider when deciding if you should lose more weight.

❖ Are you strength training? Muscle weighs more than fat but looks a heck of a lot better.
❖ Where's the weight? If those stubborn pounds are around your middle, they could be increasing your risk of heart disease, diabetes, and even some types of cancer. Waist measurements greater than 39 inches for women younger than 40, greater than 35 inches for women 40 or older, and greater than 33 inches for postmenopausal women pose greater health risks.
❖ Do you have any signs of high cholesterol, high blood pressure, or high blood glucose? These may be the first clues that your weight is affecting your health.
❖ Is it realistic to eat any less or to exercise any more? "You can't diet forever," Dr. Levitsky says. "It's better to choose a lifestyle that encourages healthy weight by making exercise and healthy eating a regular part of the program than to obsess over a few pounds."

23

Stop Feeding Your Emotions

Can't stick with a weight-loss plan? There may be a hidden connection between your mood and your eating habits. Read through the following situations and decide whether any of them sound familiar.

❖ You and your husband have an argument about the credit card bill. You leave the house in a huff and end up dining alone. Does being vexed give you a voracious appetite?

❖ Your five-year-old is finally resting quietly after a bad fall. Do you raid the cupboards for some "pain relief" of your own?

❖ You're home alone on a Saturday night. Do you dish up some cobbler à la mode to keep you company?

❖ Someone very close to you dies suddenly. Does your grief spur you to eat more than you normally would?

❖ You've earned an unexpected $200 bonus at work. Do you and your co-workers celebrate with a five-course meal at your favorite restaurant?

If you answered yes to any of the questions above, then how you feel is influencing how you eat—at least some of the time. "Many of us use food to satisfy our emotional needs as well as our physical needs," says Peter Miller, Ph.D., executive director of the Hilton Head Health Institute in South Carolina. "So the way we feel often dictates what—and how much—we eat."

In fact, Dr. Miller estimates that as much as half of our food consumption is emotionally driven. Which means that we're eating twice as much as our bodies need. And all of that extra is stored as—you guessed it—fat.

Fortunately, you don't have to remain at the emotional mercy of food. This chapter will help you identify how much of your eating is tied to your feelings—and what you can do about it.

If Anger Is Your Trigger . . .

Anger fuels the appetite in three ways. If you feel that you've been wronged, you may overeat to gain compensation. If you're mad at yourself—say, for cheating on your diet—you may overeat to punish yourself subconsciously. If you're upset with a loved one, you may overeat to release your rage.

"Women are socialized to suppress 'masculine' emotions such as anger," says George Parks, Ph.D., a counselor in private practice in Seattle who specializes in addictive behaviors. What's worse, we're seldom taught ways of dealing with our suppressed emotions, so we eat as a means of coping.

What does Dr. Parks suggest? Confront the source of your ire. Voice your feelings of frustration. Release the anger that tends to fuel french-fry frenzies and barbecue-chip binges by addressing the issue head-on.

If Anxiety Whets Your Appetite . . .

Anxiety manifests itself in two distinct forms: specific (you're concerned about a particular event, such as your child's first trip to overnight camp) and general (you're constantly worried about things that might happen). And—surprise, surprise—both can trigger overeating.

Research suggests that some anxiety-ridden overeaters binge in an effort to medicate themselves. The theory: Carbohydrate-rich foods such as cookies and cake boost the level of serotonin, a brain chemical that produces a calming effect.

To help you calm down without the calories, John Foreyt, Ph.D., director of the Behavioral Medicine Research Center at Baylor College of Medicine in Houston, offers these helpful tips.

❖ Look for patterns in your behavior. For instance, do you reach for snack cakes whenever your in-laws are coming for a visit? Once you've found the source of your anxiety, you can take steps to change the situation that troubles you.

❖ Quiz yourself when a craving strikes. Ask yourself, "Am I really hungry? If not, why am I thinking of eating? How will I feel if I don't eat?" Odds are, eating won't make you feel better about the situation—just guilty about feeding your face.

❖ To soothe your nerves and take your mind off the strawberry cheesecake in your freezer, sit in a chair with your eyes closed. Breathe easily and regularly as you empty your mind. Then concentrate on tensing and relaxing each part of your body, beginning with your toes and finishing with your forehead. After 10 to 20 minutes of this, your anxiety should dissipate, if not disappear.

❖ Get a good night's sleep. Researchers have found that well-rested people are less anxious and better able to resist the urge to overeat.

If Boredom Gets You Bingeing . . .

You can't find one show to watch on your TV's 57-plus channels. And you don't have the energy for an hour-long phone conversation with your best friend. So you do what just about any incredibly bored person would do: Reach for the hot-fudge ripple ice cream.

Boredom is one of the most common excuses people give for overeating. So it's fitting that the remedy is one of the most straightforward: diversion. "I encourage my patients to take classes and become involved in something they enjoy, be it experimenting with low-fat cooking or volunteering at a hospital," says Dr. Foreyt. A few other ways to spend your time: Participate in a favorite sport, read a trashy novel, shop early for holiday gifts, play with your pets, rearrange your closets, take in a movie, or give yourself an at-home spa treatment.

Of course, when a snack attack hits, time is of the essence. You have to occupy yourself immediately, or you risk giving in. Keep yourself busy for at least 10 minutes.

If Depression Leads to Dining . . .

First of all, there's a big difference between "the blues" and genuine clinical depression. To determine which is the cause of your bingeing, ask yourself these questions.

❖ Do you feel as though your eating is out of control?
❖ Do you fear that you can't stop when you want to?
❖ Do you spend an excessive amount of time thinking about food—when and what you're going to eat next and how much you're going to overeat?
❖ Do you often feel bad about yourself, as though you're no longer a "good" person?
❖ Do you frequently feel as though the future looks grim?

If you answer yes to all of these questions, you may be suffering from clinical depression. It's very treatable—but also very serious. So see your doctor pronto.

If you answer no even once, however, chances are that you're simply experiencing the blues. "Dispirited eaters attempt to inject pleasure and satisfaction into their lives through food," says Ronald Podell, M.D., director of the Center for Bio-Behavioral Psychiatry in Los Angeles and author of *Contagious Emotions*. Problem is, these folks often feel more depressed after they eat—when the postbinge guilt hits—than they did beforehand. This pattern can lead to more eating, bluer blues, and ever-diminishing self-esteem.

To combat the blues without food, find a sympathetic ear—a relative, friend, or acquaintance with whom you can talk over your problem. "Reach for the phone rather than the fridge," urges Dr. Podell. "By sharing your feelings, you'll be less likely to self-medicate with food."

You might also try getting active. "In addition to burning calories, exercise stimulates the production of brain chemicals that have a soothing effect and promote a sense of well-being," says Dr. Foreyt. Working out three to five times a week for at least 30 minutes per session helps keep the basic blues at bay.

Is Your Family Sabotaging Your Diet?

You're doing your darnedest to lose weight. You're sticking with a smart eating plan. You're walking every day, and you feel good about it. Now if only your family could muster a little support for your efforts.

For some strange reason, instead of getting behind you, they seem bent on tripping you up. Your husband brings home take-out pizza with double cheese for dinner. Your kids wrap themselves around your ankles as you inch toward the door with your gym bag. And even after you've managed to drop a dress size, no one utters a peep of praise.

Lack of support on the home front is a common experience among those undertaking a weight-loss program, experts say. What's going on? It could be that your commitment to change poses a threat to those closest to you, says Joyce Nash, Ph.D., a San Francisco–based clinical psychologist specializing in eating disorders and author of *The New Maximize Your Body Potential: Lifetime Skills to Successful Weight Management.*

Maybe your husband also needs to lose weight but doesn't want to, Dr. Nash notes. Or perhaps your family is confused because you're sending mixed signals. You say you want to lose weight, but you suffer every step of the way. So your loved ones think they're being helpful by offering you treats and excuses—in a sense rescuing you from the tortures of your endeavor.

In most cases, family members aren't aware that their actions and words may be undermining your efforts. But whether it's on purpose or not, sabotage is something you have to tackle head-on if you want to succeed, says exercise physiologist Jennifer Bolger, fitness program director of the Mission Valley YMCA in San Diego and creator of the Y's 12-week program for people learning to exercise on a regular basis. The bottom line is that if you don't have social support for your efforts, your chances for success are almost nil.

Identifying the Enemy

Following are profiles of some of the most common weight-loss saboteurs. Do you recognize any of them in your own family? If so, read on for advice on how to win them over to your side.

The "Oops, Are Those My Chips?" Saboteur. Your kids leave junk food strewn in your path.

Winning them over: Teenagers in particular have a talent for leaving bags of potato chips lying on the coffee table, says Dr. Nash. She suggests trying a little reverse psychology. Instead of yelling at them, say something like, "I'd really appreciate your help in my efforts to lose weight. It would be great if you

All in the Family

Where does your family weigh in on the support-to-sabotage scale?

Suppose you were to tell your husband and kids that you're planning to lose 15 pounds by switching to a low-fat diet and working out vigorously three times a week. How would they respond?

A. They'd jump up and down for joy, thrilled at the prospect of not having to eat french fries and ice cream anymore. They'd beg to sign up for aerobics classes with you. They'd also start planning and saving, so they could treat you to a celebratory cruise when you reach your weight-loss goal.

B. Your husband would say, "That's nice, honey. Let me know if there's anything I can do, as long as I don't have to eat differently and you don't expect me to set foot in a health club or otherwise break a sweat." Meanwhile, your kids would go about their lives as if they hadn't heard you.

C. Everyone would groan in unison, "But what about Friday nights at the all-you-can-eat Beef and Butter buffet? And does this mean that you're going to quit looking for the closest parking space at the video store and that we'll always have to take the stairs at the mall?"

D. They'd simultaneously burst into laughter. "Oh sure, Mom," they'd say. "That's a good one. Now let's go to Grubby Greaseburger's Fried Food Emporium to celebrate."

Okay, you get the picture. Chances are that your family is not quite as bad as B, C, or D but not nearly as good as A. Fortunately, you can change their saboteur ways.

---

wouldn't leave chips lying around." If the behavior comes up again, keep your response light: "Whoops! I bet you forgot about these potato chips. Would you mind taking them out of my sight right now?" Kids are much more likely to cooperate if you approach them in a nice manner, notes Dr. Nash.

The "I Love You as You Are" Saboteur. Your husband tells you that he thinks you look great carrying a few extra pounds, which makes you wonder if you're doing the right thing by trying to slim down.

Winning him over: Maybe he's for real, or maybe he's threatened by the prospect of your losing weight and looking attractive to other men, says Dr. Nash. You need to decide what you want, then convey that message to your spouse.

"I took a good look at myself in the mirror and thought about how I felt in my body," recalls Joan D'Amato, whose husband claimed he liked her plump. "I ended up telling him, 'I appreciate your saying that I don't have to lose weight, but to tell you the truth, I'd feel a lot better a few pounds lighter.'" She has since lost 10 pounds, and her husband isn't complaining. Chances are that yours won't either.

The "It's All about Me" Saboteur. Your hubby and kids turn up their noses at your healthy, low-fat meals and expect you to fix separate "nondiet" meals for them.

Winning them over: For starters, know that as a wife and mom, you're not obligated to always take care of everyone else. "Although you have duties, you also have rights—including the right to take good care of yourself," says Dr. Nash.

Making separate meals is unrealistic and exhausting. Don't do it. Explain to your family that it's very important for you to cut calories. Try to cook meals that everyone can enjoy. And tell them that they can "undiet" your cooking with condiments, if they wish. At dinnertime, for instance, your kids can butter up their baked potatoes while you eat yours with chives. Or you can adapt a family meal by eating less of the main course and more salad.

You can also "sneak" healthier meals into your diet, according to Ellie Krieger, R.D., a nutritionist in private practice in New York City. "Prepare fresh vegetables without saying a word about the fact that they're steamed and fat-free. Or try cutting out half of the meat in chili or half of the cheese in lasagna." Another trick: Get your kids involved in helping you cook. It'll whet their appetites for the meal.

If your family continues to give you a hard time, you need to get tough. You may have to say, "I'm not cooking separate meals, and that's that. Here's what the dinner menu will be for the next week. If you don't like it, please make other arrangements."

The "Boob-Tube Snacker" Saboteur. Every night, your husband sits in front of the television wolfing down snacks.

Winning him over: "This is really common and really difficult to put a stop to," says Krieger. "Maybe your munching has been a couple's activity. Now only he's allowed to snack, but you're so tempted." Try inviting your husband to join in an alternative nighttime activity, such as taking a walk after dinner. If he can't be diverted from his TV chow-down session, let it be. "It's important to recognize that he's making his choice and you're making yours, and that's fine," says Krieger.

Meanwhile, you can change your TV-snacking ways by enjoying a glass of sparkling mineral water, clanking with ice cubes and topped with a twist of lime. Or brew and savor a cup of delicious herbal tea. "Honestly, you can get used to watching TV and not eating," says Krieger. "It takes time to change a habit, but you can do it."

The "Bag o' Goodies" Saboteur. Your husband and kids bring home fattening treats.

Winning them over: "Your family may see you struggling to lose weight and think that they're making you feel better by offering you sweet temptations," says Dr. Nash. "Your mouth is telling them 'no, no, no,' but your eyes are saying 'yes, yes, yes.' They want to rescue you."

Make it clear to everyone that you don't want food around that can wreak havoc with your weight-loss goals. In some cases, words alone may not suffice. The husband of one of Dr. Nash's patients brought home candy whenever his wife went on a diet. When she started a new weight-loss effort right before Easter, he walked in the house with a gift-wrapped giant chocolate egg. His wife thanked him, then cut the candy into bite-size pieces as he watched, dumbstruck. She proceeded to grind the pieces to bits in the garbage disposal. "That was the last time he ever brought candy home," says Dr. Nash.

The "Out to Lunch" Saboteur. Your family complains that you won't go to fast-food joints or favorite restaurants with them.

Winning them over: This problem has to be worked out together. The husband of one of Dr. Nash's patients insisted that his wife keep going to McDonald's with him. In a joint therapy session, the woman told her husband how important it was to her to steer clear of high-fat fast food. The husband admitted that his real gripe was that he didn't want to lose weight or be deprived. They agreed that he could still go to fast-food restaurants—but he'd have to do so without her.

Some family members may accuse you of not being fun anymore if, say, you refuse to go to their favorite fried-chicken place. In that case, Krieger suggests trying to come up with a fun alternative. Maybe suggest going to another fast-food restaurant that has really good rotisserie chicken. And consider this: If you've been eating healthfully all week, you can probably afford to join your family at the fried-chicken place as long as you limit yourself to one piece of chicken and two low-calorie side dishes.

The "Guilt Trip" Saboteur. Your husband and kids make you feel guilty about spending time exercising instead of being with them.

Winning them over: "Many women come to our program feeling guilty about leaving their families for an hour or two," says Bolger. "They think 'I don't see my kids enough as it is.' A lot of times a woman's family can handle it just fine, but her guilt is still getting in the way."

In situations like this, Bolger recommends a technique that she calls positive reorientation. Here's how it works: Instead of feeling guilty about not being with your kids, tell yourself that because you're doing something great for yourself, you're being a better mom. You're setting a good example by showing your kids that exercise is an important part of a healthy lifestyle.

As for a forlorn husband, try enticing him into exercising with you. "Having an exercise partner is always a big motivational boost," notes Bolger. "And having your spouse as your partner adds to your list of shared interests while enhancing your fitness."

The "I Didn't Authorize This" Saboteur. Your family acts confused when you head toward the door for your workout.

Winning them over: The problem may simply be one of scheduling. Your husband says fine to your exercise program, then balks when he realizes that it conflicts with his poker night and that you won't be available to watch the kids.

Schedule your exercise sessions, urges Bolger. Sit down with the whole family, calendar in hand, and negotiate days and details. Get it down to something like "On Mondays and Wednesdays, I'd like to go to the gym. So can you be responsible for making dinner and getting the kids bathed and ready for bed? I'd really appreciate it."

The "Drill Sergeant" Saboteur. Your avid-exerciser husband tells you that you're not working out often enough or hard enough.

Winning him over: Lynn Bragin's husband, who bikes every day and is a serious weight lifter, apparently thought his armchair coaching was helping her. But in fact, she found being told that her exercise program wasn't up to par demoralizing.

"We hear this from a number of new exercisers," says Bolger. "The best approach is to go home armed with the research that indicates more isn't better. Recent studies show that for long-term fitness and weight maintenance, it's not necessary to do three sets of a strength-training exercise instead of one."

"I ended up having to tell my husband things like 'It's great that you can cycle that much and lift all that weight, but that's not my goal,'" says Bragin. "I'm doing my best, and this is enough for me."

The "Whaddaya Mean You Lost Weight?" Saboteur. Your family never says a word about your obvious weight-loss success.

Winning them over: Offering praise and encouragement doesn't come naturally to everyone. Accept this about your family. Then train them to change.

Laura Baxter, who has lost both weight and inches on her weight-loss program, says of her husband: "It's not that he discourages me. He just doesn't think to tell me that I look good." Her strategy is to report to him on her progress and to ask point-blank for feedback. "I tell him how much weight I've lost, then ask him how I look. 'Fantastic,' he'll say. A lot of men—and he's one of them—just don't get it. We want them to notice."

You may even have to put the exact words you want to hear into their mouths, according to Bolger. Say to your kids, "Please tell me 'Gee, we're proud of you, Mom,' not just 'Gee, we sure miss you while you're at the gym.'"

Nutrition Know-How

Quick Quiz

Are You Eating Right?

What follows is a rundown of the subtle signals your body may send when your eating habits could use some tweaking. Begin by marking each statement "yes" or "no." Then for each yes response, refer to the next section to find out what your symptom means and what nutritional changes may correct it. *Note:* Some of these symptoms can indicate a more serious health problem. So if they don't go away after you change your eating habits, see your doctor.

_____1. Your skin is a wasteland—dry, itchy, scaly.

_____2. Your hair has lost its shine.

_____3. You're constipated more often than not.

_____4. You have gas more frequently than you used to.

_____5. Your joints creak.

_____6. Your gums hurt like crazy.

_____7. Your bones break.

_____8. You've forgotten why you started reading this article.

What Your Yes Means

1. Skin that is borderline reptilian not just in winter but year-round may signal a vitamin A deficiency.

What you can do: Every time you go to the supermarket, make sure that your basket contains at least two orange-yellow and two dark green fruits or vegetables. Spinach, broccoli, apricots, cantaloupes, carrots, and sweet potatoes all have enough vitamin A to keep you from looking like a lizard and scratching like a dog. (For sneaky ways to increase your produce consumption, see The Vegetable-Hater's Guide to Nutrition on page 184.)

2. In extreme cases, your hair can lose its luster because of a significant protein or iron deficiency, especially if you're a vegetarian or you've gone on a fad diet.

What you can do: Avoid fad diets like the plague. Invariably, any pounds that disappear will find their way back. Instead, eat nutritious low-fat foods and exercise regularly. (Turn to 101 Easiest Ways to Win at Weight Loss on page 118.) If you're a vegetarian, be sure to eat a good mix of vegetables, grains, and beans so that you take in the balanced protein you'd normally get from meats.

3. Constipation is a sign that you need more fiber in your diet.

What you can do: Aim for the Daily Value of fiber, which is 25 grams. A bowl of bran flakes at breakfast supplies about 5 grams. Mix in a handful of raisins for another 4 grams. Munch on a couple of apples or a handful of carrot sticks every afternoon, and you'll be well on your way to hitting the 25-gram mark. As you increase your fiber intake, make sure that you increase your fluid intake as well. Water and other liquids help fiber do its job. (For more information about the health benefits of water, see The Liquid You Can't Live Without on page 209.)

4. Eating too much fiber or switching to a high-fiber diet too quickly causes problems of its own. In particular, your body will produce a lot more . . . um, exhaust than it would by processing more digestible foods.

What you can do: Increase your fiber intake gradually. If you've been eating only 10 grams per day, don't suddenly increase to 25 grams per day. Add 5 grams to start, then another 5 grams after a week or so. If your gas problem comes from eating an abundance of beans and other legumes, buy yourself a bottle of Beano. This product, which is sold in grocery stores and drugstores, helps break down sugars that cause gas.

5. You may have a lack of fish in your diet. Fish such as salmon and tuna contain omega-3 fatty acids, which keep joints moving smoothly while increasing blood flow and reducing joint inflammation and pain.

What you can do: Twice a week, replace the beef or poultry in your dinner entrée with a thick salmon or tuna steak.

6. If canker sores are a constant presence, your mouth may be screaming for more acidophilus. This beneficial bacterium can help balance the natural flora that can otherwise run amok in your mouth, causing sores and other gum problems, according to Robert Wildman, Ph.D., professor of human nutrition at the University of Delaware in Newark.

What you can do: Eat a cup of yogurt every day as a snack. Look for yogurt that contains live active cultures. The label will say so.

7. Your bones may be prone to breaking because you aren't consuming enough calcium and vitamin D, your body's chief bone-builders.

What you can do: Drink a tall glass of calcium-fortified orange juice at breakfast. Add a slice of low-fat cheese to your sandwich at lunch. Eat a cup of yogurt as a mid-afternoon snack. And drink a glass of fat-free or 1 percent milk before you go to bed. (For more ways to strengthen your skeleton, see The Latest Strategies for Stronger Bones on page 64.)

8. You may not be getting enough B vitamins. Folate and vitamins B_6 and B_{12} help the brain operate at peak levels while controlling homocysteine, an amino acid that can hamper blood flow to the brain.

What you can do: Think beans of all kinds. They're the best sources of folate and vitamin B_6. Vitamin B_{12} is found in abundance in most meats and seafood.

The Vegetable-Hater's Guide to Nutrition

As kids, we were impressively creative with our tactics for evading the consumption of undesirable vegetables. Now that we're adults, we have no excuse for concealing our peas or brussels sprouts beneath lettuce-leaf garnishes. After all, we know better. Vegetables are good for us.

Still, many of us would just as soon forgo that forkful of sweet potato in favor of a fistful of potato chips. Our palates remain in a state of adolescence, rebelling against the grown-up notion of what constitutes optimum nutrition.

Sure, we can attempt to compensate for an underdeveloped diet by popping a daily multivitamin. But while that pill may provide the Daily Values of important vitamins and minerals, it lacks other substances that are essential to good health.

First on the list is phytochemicals. These little-known compounds shield vegetables from viruses, bacteria, and fungi. In humans, they offer protection from heart disease, cancer, and a variety of other debilitating conditions.

Second is fiber—you know, roughage. Unless you're swallowing your One-a-Day with a glass of Metamucil, you're not getting enough of the stuff. Yet you need fiber to keep your intestinal tract working properly. As a bonus, fiber can lower both your cholesterol level and your risk of colon cancer.

Of course, knowing the "why" behind eating vegetables doesn't necessarily help with the "how." To that end, we've devised a sneaky plan for slipping these foods into your diet so that they're virtually unnoticeable. Follow our advice closely, and you'll reap the benefits of eating vegetables without inciting a riot among your tastebuds.

Eat Minimal Produce, Get Maximum Nutrition

Pick and prepare your produce wisely, and you can eat fewer vegetables because every mouthful will be nutritionally packed. Here's how to make sure you do it right.

Bring them in from the cold. No matter how cheap it is, don't be tempted to purchase a case of fresh vegetables at the local Mega-Buy. After chilling in your fridge for a few days, most of the veggies will have lost substantial amounts of their nutrients. So unless you're going to eat them immediately, buy frozen instead.

"Vegetables are usually frozen within a few hours of harvest, so the nutritional quality can actually be better than fresh," says Diane Barrett, Ph.D., associate professor of food science and technology at the University of California,

Davis. Canned vegetables are fine if you're stocking a bomb shelter. But they tend to lack flavor, and they lose their B vitamins to the heat of the canning process.

Color-coordinate. When you're in the supermarket produce aisle, tear off one of those plastic bags and stuff it with the most brightly colored vegetables you see. Vibrant hues usually correspond with higher nutrient contents, says licensed dietitian Anne Dubner, R.D., a nutrition consultant and spokesperson for the American Dietetic Association. So go easy on iceberg lettuce, celery, and cucumbers and load up on carrots, tomatoes, red bell peppers, and sweet potatoes. Also, opt for darker shades of greens. Romaine lettuce, for example, has nearly seven times the vitamin C and twice the calcium of its paler iceberg cousin.

Discover raw power. If you want to ruin perfectly good produce, just add water. "When you cook in water, the water-soluble B and C vitamins are leached out," says Dr. Barrett. Anywhere from 33 to 90 percent of the vitamin C typically ends up at the bottom of the pot.

A 15-minute boiling will also knock out a lot of the flavor, adds Dubner. Snap peas and cauliflower are examples of vegetables that are usually served cooked but that taste better and are more nutritious raw.

Flash 'em. If you must boil your vegetables, try flash boiling instead. It's one of the fastest and healthiest ways to cook. Just bring a pot of water to a rolling boil, add your vegetables, count to 10, then drain. This technique softens the veggies a bit while preserving much of their vitamin and mineral content. Steaming and microwaving will also make produce more palatable without sapping its nutrients. "They're good cooking choices because both let you cook in a minimal amount of water," says Dr. Barrett. For variety, try stir-frying.

Disguise Your Vegetables

You probably know at least one person who loves to smother everything in ketchup. Now admittedly, broccoli with ketchup is an acquired taste. But consider the underlying principle: This person is getting the same vitamins, minerals, phytochemicals, and fiber as you, but without gagging.

If you're not quite ready to start dousing all of your least favorite vegetables with the condiment of your choice, try these tips instead.

Find a good hiding place. It's an old trick, but a good one: Chop or shred vegetables and add them to dishes that will hide their flavors. Put spinach in chili, mushrooms in macaroni and cheese, artichokes on pizza, peppers and scallions in omelets. And when you make a sandwich or burger, dress it with tomatoes, lettuce, onions, and peppers, then smother everything with ketchup, mustard, or low-fat mayonnaise. Pungent vegetables, such as onions and garlic, can be finely chopped and added to spaghetti sauce.

Create look-alikes. Cut sweet potatoes, turnips, and rutabaga into thin slices, then season them with your choice of spices and bake them as vegetable chips.

Take a dip. Store washed and cut vegetables in a resealable plastic bag in your refrigerator. (If you don't have time to prep the produce yourself, look for precut veggies in your supermarket.) When you want a snack, skip the nachos and instead dip the vegetables in salsa. Or use low-fat onion dip, low-fat cheese spread, or your favorite salad dressing. Some of the best veggie dippers are sugar snap peas, carrot sticks, sweet pepper wedges, and broccoli florets.

If All Else Fails . . .

The following strategies target the hard-core vegetable hater. They're meant as a last resort, when nothing else makes produce more pleasing to your palate.

Sip your nutrients. Buy a vegetable juice such as V-8. "Some of the water may be removed in the juicing process, so you could end up with more concentrated forms of the nutrients in the vegetables," explains Dr. Barrett. On the downside, juices usually don't have as much fiber as whole vegetables.

If you can't stomach traditional carrot and tomato juices, try V-8 Splash. It contains 25 percent fruit juice (apple, pineapple, kiwi, lime, and mango), which covers up the carrot flavor. Or make a nonalcoholic Bloody Mary for breakfast: Add Worcestershire sauce, hot-pepper sauce, a squeeze of lemon or lime, and maybe some horseradish to your juice. Garnish with celery.

Fill up on fruits. You've reached the point of absolute surrender. Accept the fact that you'll never eat enough vegetables and then start adding more fruits to your diet. "Fruits provide most of the same vitamins and minerals as vegetables," says Leslie Bonci, R.D., a dietitian at the University of Pittsburgh. And no, raspberry ice cream doesn't count.

Smart Picks in the Supermarket

Which is healthier, cola or apple juice?

Okay, so that's a no-brainer. How about apple juice or orange juice?

Hmmm . . . That has you thinking, doesn't it?

You'll find out the answer a bit later in this chapter. The point is, you probably deal with many such "food face-offs"—Butter or margarine? Ice cream or frozen yogurt? Olive oil or corn oil?—on a typical visit to the supermarket. In many instances, the healthier choice is not crystal-clear, so price or taste, not nutrition, may dictate what you buy.

To help make your food shopping a little easier, Liz Applegate, Ph.D., a nutrition lecturer at the University of California, Davis, has analyzed eight popular food matchups. For each pair, she has outlined the nutritional facts that you should consider when making your choice. When appropriate, she has named a "winner."

Butter versus Margarine

This may be the longest-running food debate of all time, with no resolution in sight. Early on, margarine seemed the way to go because butter contains saturated fat. Then along came studies showing that the trans fats in margarine

Margarine: Down for the Count?

For years, researchers have suspected that trans fats—the kind of fat found in margarine—contribute to heart disease by raising "bad" low-density lipoprotein (LDL) cholesterol and depleting "good" high-density lipoprotein (HDL) cholesterol. An analysis of data from the Framingham Heart Study—the landmark long-term study that tracked the health of residents of Framingham, Massachusetts—seems to confirm the researchers' suspicions.

Among more than 800 of the study's participants, the rate of heart disease among those who ate at least five teaspoons of margarine per day was almost twice that of those who ate none. The correlation stuck even when other risk factors—including age, fat intake, and activity level—were taken into account.

According to Matthew Gillman, the Harvard Medical School epidemiologist who conducted the analysis, the findings raise concern because trans fats permeate the American diet. They're found not only in margarine but also in foods made with hydrogenated vegetable oil. (Hydrogenation is the process used to harden liquid vegetable oil.)

Until scientists have an opportunity to further investigate trans fats, your best bet is to steer clear of them. If you prefer margarine to butter, choose the tub or liquid variety. Both tend to have fewer trans fats than stick margarine. Also, go easy on fast foods and prepared baked goods. About 75 percent of trans fats in the typical American diet come from sources such as these.

HEALTH FLASH

are just as bad as saturated fat. Trans fats form during hydrogenation, the chemical process that converts a liquid oil to a solid stick or tub of margarine.

Both butter and margarine are pure fat. A tablespoon of butter contains 12 grams of fat, including 8 grams of saturated fat, as well as a small amount of cholesterol. Research suggests that the type of saturated fat in butter, called stearic acid, may not raise blood cholesterol as much as other types of saturated fat.

Margarine matches butter in terms of total grams of fat, but a tablespoon has just two grams of saturated fat. Plus, margarine contains no cholesterol. That's the good news. The bad news is that most margarines have one to two grams of trans fats per tablespoon. Trans fats may raise blood cholesterol levels.

The winner: Too close to call. Your best bet is to use each sparingly, thus keeping your total fat and cholesterol intakes to a minimum.

Wheat Bread versus 100 Percent Whole-Wheat Bread

Both types supply 140 calories and two grams of fat per two slices. But wheat bread is made with refined wheat flour (you'll see it mentioned in the ingredients list). For this reason, it contains less fiber than 100 percent whole-wheat bread—two to three grams compared with four to five grams per two slices. Plus, 100 percent whole-wheat bread contains extra minerals such as chromium and zinc as well as vitamin B_6 and folate. All of these exist in only trace amounts in wheat bread because the germ and other nutrition-packed parts of the grain are removed during processing.

The winner: 100 percent whole-wheat bread, no matter how you slice it. Look for 100 percent whole-wheat bagels, pastas, and cereals, too.

Beef or Pork Hot Dogs versus Turkey Hot Dogs

Depending on the brand and size, each type supplies between 140 and 200 calories. Turkey dogs usually have about 40 fewer calories than traditional dogs, but don't let this entice you too much. Both get more than two-thirds of their calories from fat, and both pack more than 500 milligrams of sodium—about 20 percent of your daily limit and a big concern if you're battling high blood pressure. Neither is a great source of protein, with only about six grams per hot dog. That's roughly equal to the amount in two slices of bread.

The winner: Another tie, although turkey dogs may have a slight edge based on their lower calorie content. If you do eat a hot dog, try to combine it with vegetarian baked beans and a fruit salad for extra protein, fiber, vitamins, and minerals.

Apple Juice versus Orange Juice

These two heavyweights of the juice world both contain up to 120 carbohydrate calories per eight ounces. That's why they're great choices to quench your thirst after a workout. If you're looking for vitamins and minerals, however, go with orange juice. An eight-ounce glass of apple juice supplies a mere 2 percent of the Daily Value (DV) for several B vitamins and just 14 percent of the DV for potassium. By comparison, an eight-ounce glass of orange juice supplies 170 percent of the DV for vitamin C, almost 60 percent of the DV for folate, and 25 percent of the DV for potassium.

The winner: Orange juice. For extra fiber and cancer-fighting phytochemicals called flavonoids, eat whole oranges, too.

Ice Cream versus Frozen Yogurt

You may have ditched ice cream for frozen yogurt in hopes of cutting your fat intake. But unless you pick a low-fat or nonfat product, frozen yogurt has about the same fat content as ice cream. Still, both supply about 25 percent of your daily calcium quota and about 5 grams of protein per cup. Not bad for a dessert.

The winner: A toss-up. Whichever way you go, pick a nonfat or low-fat variety—and limit yourself to one serving per sitting.

Olive Oil versus Corn Oil

This is the matchup that people seem to have the most questions about. Olive oil and corn oil supply the same number of calories, all of them from fat. But the type of fat differs dramatically.

Olive oil contains mostly cholesterol-lowering monounsaturated fat and a small amount of polyunsaturated fat, otherwise known as linoleic acid. Linoleic acid is essential for good health, although you need only about a teaspoon daily.

Corn oil contains very little monounsaturated fat, but it's loaded with linoleic acid—probably more than you need. Research has shown that a diet rich in linoleic acid may lower your total cholesterol, which is good. But in the process, it may also lower your "good" high-density lipoprotein (HDL) cholesterol, which is bad.

The winner: Olive oil, for its monounsaturated fat.

Don't Be a Bottom Feeder

Fruit is good for you. So yogurt with fruit in it must be good for you, too. Right?

Not necessarily.

For the most nutritious yogurt, skip the varieties with fruit on the bottom, advises Sheldon Margen, M.D., professor emeritus of public health at the University of California, Berkeley. The "fruit" may be mostly jam, which packs the equivalent of eight to nine teaspoons of sugar per cup—nearly as much as a can of soda. Instead, choose plain nonfat yogurt and add your own berries, suggests Dr. Margen. Or stick with flavors such as lemon, which don't contain fruit.

Eggs versus Fat-Free Egg Substitutes

Egg substitutes have become popular among those who are worried about their fat and cholesterol intakes (virtually all of us, in other words). It's true that an egg supplies about five grams of fat and about 70 percent of an entire day's cholesterol quota. But unless you've been cautioned about your cholesterol level by your doctor, eggs can be a legitimate (albeit small) part of a healthful diet. One egg provides 25 percent of the DV for vitamin B_{12} and about 10 percent of the DVs for folate, riboflavin, vitamin A, and vitamin D. Fat-free egg substitutes contain smaller amounts of these nutrients.

The winner: Eggs, unless you've been told to cut back on dietary cholesterol. If you have, use fat-free egg substitute to make an omelet, then stuff it with nutrient-rich vegetables.

Hamburgers versus Veggie Burgers

The big difference here is fat: Hamburgers have lots of it, and veggie burgers don't. Most beef patties contain 20 to 30 grams of fat, depending on the leanness of the meat. By comparison, veggie patties made with soy protein contain 0 to 10 grams of fat. Once you dress it up with condiments, a hamburger packs about 450 calories; a veggie burger has about 225.

Of course, a hamburger also has significantly larger amounts of minerals. It provides about 40 percent of the DV for iron and about 30 percent of the DV for zinc. And since vitamin B_{12} is found only in animal products, you'll miss out on it completely when you eat a veggie burger, unless it has been fortified. (The label will say so.)

Not to be outdone, the soy in veggie burgers has health benefits of its own. A high-soy diet has been linked to lower risks of heart disease, cancer, and menopausal hot flashes.

The winner: On the basis of fat content alone, the veggie burger gets the nod. To make up for the iron and zinc that you'll be missing, add plenty of beans, whole grains, and breakfast cereals to your diet.

What to Eat When You're Sick

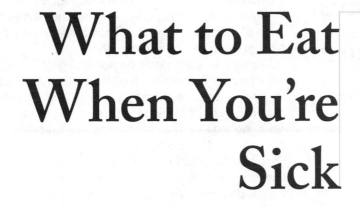

C an certain foods actually make you feel better when you're under the weather? Or is the notion that, say, a bowl of chicken soup can perk you up nothing more than a bunch of sentimental hooey?

Experts may forever debate the merits of chicken soup, but they agree on one thing: The right foods can indeed help speed recovery from a wide range of illness and injury, from a bruised leg to a bruising headache. "Nutrition is extremely important during recovery from an illness," says Jane Lanzillotti, R.D., nutrition education manager at South Shore Hospital in the Boston area. "It may not work miracles, but it can certainly help."

It's worth noting that the primary nutrient experts mention—no matter the ailment—is plain old water. Guzzling plenty of H_2O just may be the most important thing you can do not only to keep your body in good repair but also to mend it.

That said, here are nutrition prescriptions for six common health complaints.

Caught in a Cold's Grip

Forget the decongestants, suppressants, and assorted other "-ants" that line your drugstore's shelves. When you feel a cold coming on, pick up some grape-

Industrial-Strength Nutrition

Spurred by the success of low-fat everything, food manufacturers are racing to bring out the next generation of wellness products: foods that not only help prevent diseases but also treat them.

Eyeing the latest nutrition research and the aging baby boomer generation, food companies are investing enormous sums of money in what they're calling medical foods, functional foods, or nutraceuticals. Take Kellogg's. The food manufacturer recently opened the $75 million W. K. Kellogg Institute for Food and Nutrition Research to cook up cholesterol-lowering cereals and other fare for its Functional Foods division. Meanwhile, Campbell's Soup has sunk a reported $25 million to $30 million into three clinical trials of Intelligent Quisine, a line of prepared, home-delivered meals targeting consumers who have high cholesterol, high blood pressure, or diabetes.

How effective are these foods? Most are still in development, but Campbell's IQ is already out of the gate. It was designed to meet the dietary recommendations of the American Heart Association and the American Diabetes Association, then tested on 800 patients at eight university medical centers. The findings: Of those who ate IQ for 10 weeks, 73 percent reduced their cholesterol by an average of 5.5 percent; 75 percent lowered their blood pressure by an average of 4.7 percent; and 62 percent reduced their blood sugar by an average of 9.9 percent.

Some nutrition experts greet these findings warily. "In general, a diet of processed food is not the best way to eat, even if you can demonstrate that it may lower cholesterol or blood pressure," says David Schardt, associate nutritionist at the Center for Science in the Public Interest in Washington, D.C. "There are hundreds of important compounds in fruits, vegetables, grains, and beans that may be beneficial to your health. In general, the more processed a food becomes, the fewer nutrients it tends to have."

You're bound to hear more about these engineered foods in years to come. In the meantime, if you have high cholesterol, high blood pressure, or diabetes, the best diet for you is one that's loaded with whole grains and fresh fruits and vegetables but that has very little fat.

HEALTH FLASH

fruit instead. "The first thing you should do is eat a lot of foods rich in vitamin C," says Laima Wesson, R.D., health educator/dietitian for the student health service at the University of California, Los Angeles. "It's an antioxidant that helps strengthen your immune system." Citrus fruits and juices fit the bill here, as do red bell peppers, broccoli, and strawberries.

If your cold has sapped your appetite, however, you can recharge your batteries with an easy-to-digest meal—maybe a baked potato and a steaming bowl of soup. "Soups, especially tomato and vegetable soups, tend to be very rich in vitamin C," notes Kristine Clark, R.D., Ph.D., director of sports nutrition for the Center for Sports Medicine at Pennsylvania State University in University Park. "They are a very palatable way of delivering nutrients."

And if you're a big fan of milk, don't feel you have to give it up until your cold passes. "While some people—especially those with chronic asthma or other lung problems—report that drinking milk worsens their conditions, there's little in the scientific literature to indicate that milk promotes mucus," says Lanzillotti.

Beat the Runs

Your dinner not only didn't agree with you, it started a revolt in your gut. Now you have a classic case of diarrhea. Just follow three simple nutritional rules. First, drink lots of water, since it's likely you'll be dehydrated. Second, feed your body, since it's likely starved for calories. Third, avoid foods high in fiber and fat, since both substances are hard to digest. The last thing you want to do now is make your gastrointestinal tract work harder than it has to, says Paul Lachance, Ph.D., professor of food science at Rutgers University in New Brunswick, New Jersey. So avoid the raw vegetables and bran flakes, the french fries and cheesecake. Instead, go for toast with jelly or a baked potato with cottage cheese—whatever goes down easily.

If you're taking drugs to ease your digestive distress, extra precautions may be in order, says Lanzillotti. "Some antibiotics kill both the bad bacteria that make you sick and the good bacteria that allow your digestive system to function," she explains. "Eating yogurt with active cultures can help replenish these healthy bacteria." (Check the label to see whether your yogurt has active, live cultures.)

Black and Blue and Sore All Over

You've probably had your share of bumps and bruises, scrapes and sprains in your lifetime. Certainly, when such mishaps occur, a little first-aid can do a world of good. But you may not realize that eating the right foods can also help your injury heal faster.

In the case of a muscle tear or strain, go for a high-carbohydrate, moderate-protein diet, advises Susan Kleiner, R.D., Ph.D., a nutritionist based in Seattle. That means plenty of grains, beans, fruits, and vegetables. Choose a colorful mix of orange and dark green leafy vegetables as well as a variety of citrus fruits, she suggests. They'll provide antioxidants, which are important for repairing the cellular damage that occurs in a muscle tear. Also, Dr. Kleiner notes, the antioxidant vitamin E may help reduce inflammation. Good sources of vitamin E include wheat germ and vegetable oils.

If you're dealing with a cut or scrape, indulge in a few helpings of lean meat, says Thomas Alt, M.D., a cosmetic surgeon in Minneapolis who has studied nutrition's role in wound healing. "Meat is one of the best sources of the essential amino acids, which are the basic building blocks for healing," he says. "Without them, you won't heal as well or as rapidly as normal."

And if your injury is serious enough to keep you off your feet, start watching your calorie intake, cautions Mel Williams, Ph.D., professor emeritus of exercise science at Old Dominion University in Norfolk, Virginia. "If you're used to exercising, you'll have to cut your normal caloric intake to avoid putting on weight," he says.

Where, Oh Where, Has Your Energy Gone?

The good part about shuffling out of the office at 9:00 P.M. is that you can easily find your car in the parking lot. The bad part, of course, is that you probably feel chewed up and spit out. What you need is some relaxation. And what you eat—or avoid eating—can make a big difference.

"When you're working late, the last thing you want is caffeine or anything else that will prevent you from sleeping," says Heidi Shutrump, R.D., a licensed dietitian and associate director of nutrition and dietetics at Ohio State University Medical Center in Columbus. "This means avoiding chocolate, caffeinated soft drinks, even iced tea."

Instead, when you finally arrive home, curl up with carbohydrates such as bread, a bagel, pretzels, or unsweetened cereal. Carbohydrates raise your blood level of the hormone insulin, which increases uptake of the amino acid tryptophan. Tryptophan is then converted to serotonin, which is known to induce drowsiness. Tryptophan itself is found in high-protein foods, so add some peanut butter, a slice of turkey, or some low-fat cheese to the mix.

Master Migraine Pain

If you think that the only headache associated with food comes from persuading a five-year-old to eat brussels sprouts, think again. "Your diet can help produce a migraine, but unfortunately, it can't get rid of one," says Victor Herbert, M.D., J.D., director of the Nutrition Research Center at Mount Sinai Medical Center in New York City. So the best that food can do after you've had a migraine is to not wake the beast again.

Migraines are highly individualized. But some people get them from eating certain foods, especially those high in a compound called tyramine. The key suspects: organ meats such as liver and kidneys, fermented products such as soy sauce and yeast, wine, hot dogs, certain aged cheeses, chocolate, caffeine, and monosodium glutamate (MSG).

When You've Had One Too Many

Folk remedies for hangovers are more common than empty beer cans at a frat party—and, sadly, just about as useful. The best you can do, experts say, is drink plenty of water (since alcohol tends to dehydrate you) and weather the storm.

If you must try something, though, Dr. Lachance suggests drinking spicy V-8 vegetable juice or even a nonalcoholic Bloody Mary. Too much alcohol can create cell-damaging free radicals, he explains, and vegetable juice and tomato juice are good sources of antioxidants. (Antioxidants neutralize free radicals.) Also, the spices can help dilate blood vessels, which could speed recovery by improving blood circulation to your throbbing head.

One final note: Stay away from acetaminophen before, during, and after a night of drinking. Acetaminophen and alcohol is a dangerous combination that can lead to liver damage, says David Whitcomb, M.D., Ph.D., of the University of Pittsburgh Medical Center. "Doses of up to two grams—about four Extra-Strength Tylenol—are probably okay," he says. "But I recommend skipping it altogether if you're drinking."

Straight Talk on Supplements

They line the shelves of drugstores and health food stores like little soldiers. Some you recognize, such as vitamin E, calcium, and beta-carotene. Others have names that sound as if they're straight out of a science fiction novel: coenzyme Q_{10}, alpha-lipoic acid, blue-green algae, colloidal minerals.

As you cruise through this paradise of promised health, you have to wonder, "Which of these can really prevent disease and help me live longer?" Certainly, the possibilities are staggering. And nearly every day, you read or hear a news story touting the benefits of one supplement or another. Deciding what to buy can be incredibly confusing.

Well, the experts have weighed in on the hottest supplements on the market today. Here's what they say that you may want to pick up—and what you should leave on the shelf.

The Best of the Bunch

You eat nutritious foods and exercise regularly. You just want a little extra insurance to help keep disease at bay. Since you're unlikely to get optimal levels of all of the essential nutrients from foods alone (you'd have to eat too many calories), you're wise to think about supplementing.

In a perfect nutritional world, you would get all of your essential nutrients from the foods you eat. But who lives in a perfect world? As a result, many people take supplements as insurance. This is fine, as long as you don't become lazy about your eating habits and think that you're getting all the nutrition you need from your daily multi-vitamin.

This tendency showed itself in a study conducted by Australian researchers. For two years, two groups of people took the same amount of extra calcium daily. But one group got it from supplements, while the other group got it from powdered milk integrated into their daily diets. The researchers found that compared with those who took supplements, members of the group that got the powdered milk generally ate better and significantly decreased their fat intakes.

These findings just go to show that taking supplements sometimes makes people think that they can afford to be less concerned with proper nutrition. This is a mistake; there's no substitute for a well-balanced diet.

To start, select a good multivitamin/mineral supplement, along with separate supplements of vitamins C and E and calcium. (For dosages, see "What to Take Every Day.") Then consider adding the following minerals to your regimen. Research has shown that these nutrients have remarkable health benefits, yet they're probably in short supply in your diet.

Note: If you have a kidney problem, you should check with your doctor before taking any mineral in supplement form.

Chromium (for diabetes). Getting the Daily Value (DV) of 120 micrograms from foods alone is difficult. Even many multivitamins come up short. But chromium is absolutely vital to help your body process blood sugar (glucose) for energy. A low level of the mineral may increase your risk of Type II (non-insulin-dependent) diabetes. If you already have diabetes, studies have suggested that taking 200 to 1,000 micrograms of chromium every day can improve your symptoms. But more studies on long-term supplementation still need to be done. In the meantime, don't take more than 200 micrograms of chromium a day without first checking with your doctor.

Magnesium. Single-dose multivitamins supply no more than 100 milligrams of magnesium. And most of us don't eat the foods in which the mineral is most abundant—whole grains, soybeans, and nuts, for example—regularly enough

What to Take Every Day

No matter what the state of your health, you can benefit from taking a multivitamin/mineral supplement that contains 100 percent of the Daily Values of most essential vitamins and minerals. (No multivitamin contains them all.) Make sure the product you choose supplies the following nutrients in the specified amounts. These often get shortchanged in the typical diet, experts say.

❖ Chromium: 120 to 200 micrograms
❖ Copper: 2 milligrams
❖ Folic acid: 400 micrograms
❖ Magnesium: 100 milligrams
❖ Selenium: at least 10 micrograms
❖ Vitamin A/beta-carotene: 5,000 international units
❖ Vitamin B_6: 2 milligrams
❖ Vitamin D: 400 international units
❖ Zinc: 15 milligrams

Unless you have iron-deficiency anemia, look for a multivitamin without iron. You probably don't need extra. What's more, recent studies have linked high iron levels with increased risk of heart attack and atherosclerosis (a build-up of fatty deposits in the arteries).

In addition to a multivitamin, you'll want to take separate supplements of the following. They're not found in optimum amounts in any multi.

❖ Calcium: 500 to 1,000 milligrams
❖ Vitamin C: 500 milligrams (for maximum effectiveness, take as two 250-milligram doses spaced 12 hours apart)
❖ Vitamin E: 100 to 400 international units

to provide the DV of 400 milligrams. But magnesium is important. The diseases from which it could protect you are all killers: heart disease, high blood pressure, diabetes, and osteoporosis. It may also help relieve migraines. Aim for a total of 350 milligrams of magnesium a day from both your multivitamin and an individual supplement. More than that may cause diarrhea.

Selenium. This antioxidant is showing great promise as a cancer-fighter. One 10-year study of 1,300 people found that those who took a 200-microgram supplement daily cut their overall cancer rate by 39 percent and their rates of lung, prostate, and colon cancer by almost half. The amounts of selenium in your multivitamin and an individual supplement should add up to no more than 200 micrograms.

Pills with Potential

The following non-nutrient supplements have been grabbing headlines lately. While the preliminary research on them looks good, they're not for everyone. Many health experts want to see more studies before recommending them.

Alpha-lipoic acid. A relative newcomer to the market, alpha-lipoic acid is an antioxidant that your body normally makes on its own. It helps break down food into the energy needed by your cells. Supplementing may be helpful if you have or are at high risk for diabetes, because your metabolism—the process by which your body produces energy—is impaired. Preliminary studies suggest that alpha-lipoic acid prevents the nerve damage in the lower legs that often occurs as a result of diabetes, possibly because of its protective effect on smaller blood vessels.

In one study in which people with diabetes took alpha-lipoic acid supplements for four months, the effective dosage was 800 milligrams a day. The study participants reported no adverse effects.

Coenzyme Q_{10}. Coenzyme Q_{10} is another antioxidant manufactured by the body, where it goes by the name ubiquinone. While many healing powers are claimed for this supplement, its potential benefits presently appear to be limited to helping you if you have or are at risk for congestive heart failure, a condition in which your heart is too weak to pump blood to your lungs and the rest of your body. It may also be good for gum disease, a leading cause of tooth loss.

One study found that 150 milligrams of coenzyme Q_{10} per day had some therapeutic effects for people with congestive heart failure. (Those taking that amount were hospitalized 38 percent less than those taking placebos.) And 50 to 60 milligrams a day helped reverse gum disease.

Note: While coenzyme Q_{10} appears to be safe, congestive heart failure and gingivitis are not treat-it-yourself diseases. Both require a doctor's care.

Glucosamine and chondroitin. Your body makes glucosamine and chondroitin to help build and protect cartilage, the shock-absorbing cushion that caps the ends of your bones. Preliminary studies, mostly European, have shown that supplementing with both substances reduces pain and slows cartilage loss in osteoarthritis, the wear-and-tear kind of arthritis that causes aching, deteriorating joints. Alternative health practitioners and even some mainstream doctors have reported some success when using glucosamine and chondroitin in combination.

In a study by orthopedic surgeon Amal Das, M.D., in Hendersonville, North Carolina, "the combination was significantly effective for pain relief in people with mild to moderate arthritis, but not with severe arthritis," he says.

So far, both glucosamine and chondroitin appear to be safe. If you want to try them, you can get them either separately or as a combination. But be careful what you buy: A study conducted at the University of Maryland found a few products that contained far less glucosamine or chondroitin than their labels claimed. Two combination products that passed the study's quality tests were Cosamin DS and Joint Fuel.

Be sure to talk to your doctor before beginning supplementation. Follow the label directions for dosage and give the supplements eight weeks to work. If you don't notice any improvement in that time, stop taking them.

Questionable at Best

Some supplements remain mysteries that are yet to be explored by research. Others, based on a lack of evidence so far, aren't worth their expense. The following fall into one of these categories.

Blue-green algae. This supplement comes in more than 1,000 different strains that grow in lakes and oceans. The algae available as a supplement generally began life as pond scum. It does contain protein, B vitamins, and minerals. Still, it's leaving a lot of nutrition experts cold. You can get plenty of the same nutrients from foods and a multivitamin, notes Alan R. Gaby, M.D., professor of nutrition at Bastyr University in Seattle. There have also been reports of toxicity, contamination, and illness associated with some algae.

Chelated supplements. Chelation is simply a process that binds minerals with another substance, supposedly to enhance the minerals' absorption in the body. But actual studies proving better absorption are few. When a manufacturer labels a supplement as "chelated," it's usually just to make you think that product is better than the rest, says Dr. Gaby.

Chromium (for weight loss). Theoretically, it could work, says Priscilla Clarkson, Ph.D., health sciences dean and researcher at the University of Massachusetts in Boston. "Chromium enhances insulin action, and insulin aids fat metabolism," Dr. Clarkson explains. "That means that chromium could potentially burn fat. But that theory hasn't yet become fact." Studies showing that supplemental chromium helps take off the pounds have been weak or inconsistent.

Shark cartilage. Its proponents speculate that shark cartilage can prevent cancer by blocking the growth of blood vessels in tumors, depriving the tumors of nutrients necessary for growth. As yet, no well-controlled studies support this claim. And forming new blood vessels isn't always a bad thing, points out Dr. Gaby. It's useful when your cardiovascular system is trying to move blood around blockages, during pregnancy, or for wound healing, for example. Dr. Gaby also doubts that popular oral supplements of shark cartilage can even make it into the bloodstream, because their active ingredient is a protein that is destroyed by digestion.

For Guinea Pigs Only

Under the 1994 Dietary Supplement Health and Education Act, manufacturers don't have to prove that supplements work or that they're safe before selling them. The Food and Drug Administration (FDA) classifies these products as dietary supplements, not as drugs. By law, drugs must meet rigorous testing standards for safety and efficacy before getting FDA approval. Yet people often use supplements as if they were drugs—to prevent or treat disease. (By the way, it is illegal for a supplement label to claim to prevent or treat disease.) Don't be a guinea pig—don't self-prescribe the following products.

Colloidal supplements. Colloidal supplements sprang from the theory that minerals au naturel—combined the way you would find them in rich soil—are best for your body. You can't rely on fruits and vegetables for minerals, the theory goes, because bad farming practices have depleted the soil of nutrients. But this rationale doesn't quite hold up to scrutiny. "Your body is used to absorbing minerals from foods," says Jerald Foote, R.D., a consulting dietitian in private practice in Arvada, Colorado. Taking colloidal supplements is "like eating soil to get your minerals," he says.

What's more, colloidal supplements made from so-called good earth can come with an unwanted bonus—pollutants, lead, aluminum, or even arsenic. Although Foote believes that manufacturers have started removing these substances, he recommends giving colloidal supplements a wide berth.

DHEA. DHEA (short for dehydroepiandrosterone) is a weak male hormone that your body makes. As you get older, production declines. Some people turn to DHEA supplements to circumvent the symptoms of aging. "I've seen some noteworthy improvements in older patients' muscle mass and memory," says Dr. Gaby. "Their depression gets better, too." But DHEA is a steroid hormone, he cautions. In theory, it could increase your risk of breast cancer.

You should use DHEA supplements only if blood tests show that your own level is low, Dr. Gaby advises. And your doctor should always monitor the treatment.

Melatonin. Melatonin is a nonsteroidal hormone produced by your body.

Your pineal gland releases it in response to darkness, so it's closely linked to your sleep/wake cycle. Melatonin production slows as you age, which is why supplementation can be useful for older people who have phase-shift insomnia. This means that they often fall asleep later than they'd like, which leaves them exhausted the next day. Melatonin helps reset their body clocks to acceptable hours. It is also used to help ease jet lag.

Short-term use seems harmless so far, although some people have reported experiencing odd dreams. Regular, long-term use is not recommended.

Pregnenolone. Pregnenolone is an up-and-coming supplement that you'll be seeing more of in health food stores. It's another anti-aging hormone—a precursor of DHEA, explains Elson Haas, M.D., director of the Preventive Medical Center of Marin in San Rafael, California.

Pregnenolone improved the memory of aging rodents in one study, says Dr. Gaby. But research so far is sparse and preliminary.

What is known is that both pregnenolone and DHEA increase the levels of estrogen and testosterone in your body, which means that women could grow facial hair and men's breasts could enlarge, says Dr. Haas. "That isn't often seen with the lower amounts (5 to 10 milligrams) found in health food–store products," he adds. "It can happen, though."

Foote recommends using pregnenolone and DHEA with extreme caution. "Think of the care with which you and your doctor decide whether you should use hormone replacement therapy (HRT)," he says. "Anyone taking hormone supplements is doing HRT." For this reason, you should seek your doctor's advice when deciding whether supplementation is right for you.

Herbs That Work, Herbs That Don't

S t.-John's-wort, a natural antidepressant, is featured on the television news. Ginkgo, a memory aid, makes headlines in the newspaper. These and other herbs are the latest rage. And they're showing up everywhere—even in drugstores, right next to the vitamins.

Just what is all this stuff, anyway? Which herbs should you buy, and in what forms? Which are better for you: the tablets at 16 cents a pop or the capsules at $1.50 each?

Take heart. Almost everyone feels at least a little confused and helpless in Herbville. Americans are now spending more than $3 billion a year on herbal products. But the popularity of herbs has grown faster than scientists can research them or the Food and Drug Administration can regulate them. So how can you get good value—herbs that help, in a form that works?

Perhaps no one is better equipped to answer this question than Varro E. Tyler, Ph.D., Sc.D., professor emeritus of pharmacognosy (the study of medicinal plants) at Purdue University in West Lafayette, Indiana. Here, Dr. Tyler helps steer you through the herbal aisles, giving you the straight scoop on whether you should be buying the hottest-selling herbs—and which forms work best.

The Top 10

The following herbs have earned "most popular" status, based on sales. The question is, are they really worth buying? Dr. Tyler's answers may surprise you.

How
Sweet
It Is

If you're in search of a natural alternative to artificial sweeteners such as aspartame and saccharin, you may find what you're looking for in *Stevia rebaudiana-bertoni*. This South American herb is already in use in certain Asian countries as well as in Germany and Israel. And with good reason: Stevia has all the perks of its artificial cousins—zero calories, up to 300 times the sweetness of sugar—but none of the side effects.

Why haven't you heard more about stevia? The Food and Drug Administration has kept a fairly tight rein on the herb's approved uses. The organization says it has little reliable evidence of stevia's safety. Hopefully, additional scientific research will change that.

Someday you may see stevia listed among the ingredients in processed foods. In the meantime, if you want to give the herb a try, you can buy it in powdered form in health food stores. (Stevia has been approved for use as a food.) Try adding it to beverages—but remember that because of its intense sweetness, you don't need a lot of it.

Echinacea. Yes. Echinacea can prevent the common cold. It can also subdue cold symptoms.

Garlic. Yes. Garlic lowers cholesterol, thins the blood (which reduces your risk of heart attack and stroke), and fights bacteria like an antibiotic. It may also lower blood pressure and protect against stomach, skin, and colon cancer.

Ginkgo biloba. Yes. Ginkgo can aid blood flow to the brain, which perks up memory and concentration. It may also prevent or improve age-related vision loss and other circulatory problems. One recent study even showed that ginkgo helps Alzheimer's patients.

Goldenseal. Maybe. People commonly take goldenseal to boost their immunity. But the herb doesn't work well inside the body because it isn't absorbed. It is effective on the surface of the skin, however. Try it as a topical salve for canker sores or as a mouthwash to soothe a sore throat. Be aware that goldenseal is expensive and often adulterated.

Saw palmetto. Yes. For men, saw palmetto can relieve the symptoms of an enlarged prostate (too many nighttime bathroom visits, for one) without the side effects of normal drug treatment. These side effects can include impotence and loss of libido.

Aloe. Iffy. In its fresh, straight-from-the-plant form, aloe gel helps heal cuts and burns when spread on the skin. But soaps, creams, and lotions rarely tell you how much aloe they contain—usually very little, Dr. Tyler says. Plus, aloe breaks down with age and doesn't work. So fresh products are essential.

Some people use another part of the aloe plant, in capsule or tablet form, as a laxative. But it's strong, and Dr. Tyler doesn't recommend it.

Ginseng. Yes. Ginseng is a tonic that tunes up your body and mind and turns up your energy level. Be sure to buy the Asian or Panax variety rather than Siberian, which actually belongs to a different plant family.

Cat's claw. Probably not. The Spanish use cat's claw for everything from AIDS to tuberculosis. One variety of the plant may indeed have immunological powers, but another variety cancels them out. Both types could wind up in the capsule you buy—unless you find a product that contains no more than 0.02 percent tetracyclic alkaloids (the overpowering plant chemicals). "I'm not sure there are any products like this available in the United States, though," Dr. Tyler says.

Astragalus. Probably not. Astragalus is popular with practitioners of Ayurveda, an ancient Indian discipline popularized by best-selling author Deepak Chopra. Dr. Tyler says it has a reputation as an immune stimulant, but no substantial scientific evidence supports this use. "Plus, I don't think there are any standards to check on the reliability of products," Dr. Tyler adds.

Cayenne. Yes. The chemical capsaicin, which gives cayenne peppers their heat, can relieve pain. As an over-the-counter cream (available in drugstores), capsaicin is used for conditions such as shingles and postoperative mastectomy pain. In capsule form (available in health food stores), it can loosen mucous membranes and ease dry coughs from colds.

The Up-and-Comers

Although the herbs listed above are raking in the most money right now, three more are hot on their heels. Again Dr. Tyler answers the question: Are they worth buying?

St.-John's-wort. Yes. St.-John's-wort has been called nature's Prozac, and deservedly so. In Germany, it's the top prescription for mild depression. It has fewer side effects than synthetic antidepressants. In fact, reports on the herb's benefits are so good that the Food and Drug Administration is studying it for possible approval as a real drug (instead of a dietary supplement).

Kava-kava. Yes. Kava-kava may be the Xanax of the plant world. Like that drug, the herb can help you relax or mellow out when you're experiencing anxiety.

Grape seed extract. Yes. Grape seed extract is a mighty antioxidant. It saves cells threatened by free radicals and consequently helps protect against heart disease and cancer.

Too Good to Be True

As with medicines, certain herbs are better left on the store shelves. In fact, they probably shouldn't be on the market. The health claims made about them simply don't hold up under scientific scrutiny. Worse, some of them can actually harm you.

The following five herbs fall in the "don't bother" category.

❖ Alfalfa, for arthritis
❖ Burdock, as a blood purifier
❖ Damiana, as an aphrodisiac
❖ Mexican yam, as a progestin-like hormone replacement
❖ Suma, as a tonic

And definitely bypass these five herbs. All have properties that are potentially hazardous to humans.

❖ Coltsfoot, as a cough suppressant—it's carcinogenic
❖ Comfrey, for wound healing—it's carcinogenic
❖ Germander, for weight loss—it causes liver damage
❖ Sassafras, as a tonic—it's carcinogenic
❖ Yohimbe, as an aphrodisiac—it increases blood pressure and causes rapid heartbeat (and sometimes nausea and vomiting)

The Liquid You Can't Live Without

Seems like everybody is trying to tell you what to do these days, especially where your health is concerned. Eat this vegetable, take this supplement, do this exercise . . . blah, blah, blah. You're probably tired of hearing it. And really, who can blame you?

There is one piece of health advice that's so simple and straightforward that you can't afford not to listen up. In fact, it will probably be music to your ears. Ready?

Drink eight eight-ounce glasses of water a day.

Now, it may not seem like much. In fact, you've probably heard it before. But do you realize just how much this piddly little investment can pay off? It can boost your energy, your concentration, and the number of calories you burn. Plus, it will help you beat back colds and a host of other ailments.

Getting Your Fill

Plain water is best because it doesn't contain sugar, caffeine, or other compounds that can adversely affect your body and mind. But if you're not a big fan of *agua*, don't worry. Most forms of liquid count toward your daily eight, including juices, soups, and fresh fruits and vegetables (most are at least 75 percent water).

When Water Isn't Good Enough

Some exercise devotees prefer sports drinks to water simply because they taste better. The question is, do they enhance performance? That may depend on your level of activity.

According to the American College of Sports Medicine, water is fine for a workout lasting less than an hour. After all, the sandwich and banana that you ate for lunch should provide all of the electrolytes you'll need for an afternoon walk, run, or ride. (Electrolytes are electrically charged minerals, such as potassium and sodium, that power your heart and muscles.)

If you exercise vigorously for more than an hour a day, however, you start losing more electrolytes than you can spare. In such circumstances, a sports drink replaces the lost electrolytes—and it does so right away, when you need the minerals. A sports drink also delivers carbohydrates, which keep your blood sugar level up. This boosts your energy and delays fatigue, so you can finish your workout.

Even soda, tea, and coffee are acceptable, as long as you don't overdo them. Their downsides: The carbonated stuff makes you feel fuller, so you drink less. And caffeine acts as a diuretic, which means you're making more trips to the restroom—and all of that liquid is literally going to waste. The same is true of alcohol. So try to stick with the straight stuff as much as possible.

If consuming eight eight-ounce glasses of anything every day seems like a daunting task, these tips can help you do it.

Take your time. Spread your eight glasses evenly over the course of the day. Power-chugging your daily requirement in one sitting won't do you much good.

Make it convenient. Fill a 32-ounce bottle with chilled water first thing in the morning, then keep it by your side—whether you're at home, at work, or in transit. Take frequent sips throughout the day. This eliminates the need for trips to the refrigerator or water cooler.

Wash down your meals. Drink 16 ounces of water (or another liquid) at lunch and again at dinner. The sodium in the foods you eat will help your body retain the fluid, thereby giving you the most benefit.

Your Body Will Thank You

Meeting your H_2O quota every day takes some getting used to. But it's one of the healthiest habits you can have. Just look at what a little water can do for you.

Benefit 1: Drowns calories. Hunger is often thirst in disguise. Drinking a glass of water can help stave off cravings and hold you over until your next meal. It can also burn calories. According to Ellington Darden, Ph.D., author of *32 Days to a 32-Inch Waist*, you can drop a pound every eight weeks simply by drinking eight eight-ounce glasses of ice water a day. Your body has to expend 62 calories to warm that much ice water (at 49°F) to 98.6°F.

Benefit 2: Boosts endurance. Australian researchers monitored a small group of people during prolonged exercise to see how fluid intake affects endurance. The researchers found that the more water the study participants drank, the less glycogen they spent. (Muscles use glycogen for energy.)

Actually, sports drinks work on somewhat the same principle. If you rehydrate with a sports drink, your muscles use that rather than breaking down their own glycogen for energy, explains W. Larry Kenney, Ph.D., professor of physiology and kinesiology at Pennsylvania State University in University Park. As a result, your calves don't tire out as fast. So you're able to stick with your workout longer and boost your calorie burn even more.

Benefit 3: Beats colds. The mucus that coats your throat contains antibodies, which help trap cold viruses. But you can foil this ingenious defense if you're even minimally dehydrated, because a lack of water dries out your mucus-producing tissues, says John Rogers, M.D., professor of family and community medicine at Baylor College of Medicine in Houston.

If you do catch something, water can help you fight it. Here's what to do.

- ❖ Cough: For a wet cough, rather than grab the ever-tasty red syrup, chug a glass of water. It's the best expectorant around, according to Kenneth Lem, Pharm.D., a lecturer in clinical pharmacy at the University of California, San Francisco. Unless your doctor tells you otherwise, use an over-the-counter suppressant only for a dry cough.
- ❖ Fever: You know that spaced-out feeling you experience when you have a fever? Well, it's not from watching endless game shows. It's from dehydration, says Dr. Rogers. The amount you perspire as your fever breaks severely dehydrates your brain as well as your body, causing you to feel nauseated and generally zonked. So start sipping.

Benefit 4: Sharpens thinking. If you're exercising in hot weather, losing water as sweat can impair your concentration and reaction time. "There's no doubt that dehydration can affect your ability to make decisions," says Michael Sawka, Ph.D., chief of thermal and mountain medicine at the U.S. Army Research Institute of Environmental Medicine in Natick, Massachusetts. So if your workout leaves you feeling too tired to think, be sure to drink.

Benefit 5: Makes medicine go down easier. If certain medications—such as aspirin, ibuprofen, and antibiotics—tend to upset your stomach, be sure to wash them down with extra water. The water dilutes and disperses the medicine, so it's not strong enough to aggravate one spot. The more water you drink, the less your chances of stomach distress, says Dr. Lem.

Benefit 6: Foils flight-related fatigue. It's not only a time-zone thing. Fatigue during and after flight can result from dehydration, since the dry air on a plane can literally suck the water out of you. "People breathe harder because of the lower levels of oxygen," says Bruce Paton, M.D., clinical professor of surgery at the University of Colorado School of Medicine in Denver and president of the Wilderness Medical Society, based in Indianapolis. "Your body moisturizes the air and therefore loses water."

Drink an extra glass of water before you fly and a glass every hour that you're on the plane. Filling up on nonalcoholic, noncaffeinated drinks may help minimize your discomfort, says Dr. Paton. Put an orange and some bottled water in your carry-on bag to nibble and sip in-flight. It may mean extra visits to the restroom, but you need to stretch your legs anyway.

Benefit 7: Keeps things moving. "If you're constipated, it may be because you're not drinking enough," says Barbara Harland, Ph.D., professor of nutrition at Howard University in Washington, D.C. This is especially true if you've eaten a lot of fiber, which can't do its job unless you have enough fluid in your system to flush things through.

Conversely, if you have very soft stools or diarrhea, don't go on a water strike. Reducing your fluid intake won't firm things up, since bacteria are probably to blame. At the first sign of trouble, drink more, not less. You may want to sip a sports drink, which can restore lost nutrients, says Dr. Rogers. Also, eat bland foods such as bananas, rice, applesauce, and toast.

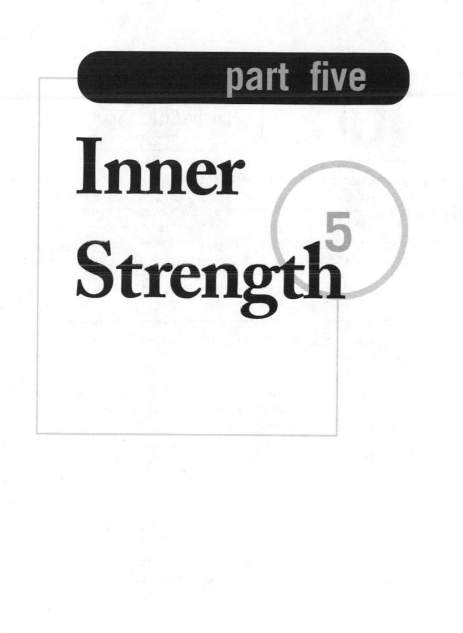

part five

Inner Strength⁵

Quick Quiz

Where Do You Stand on the Stress Scale?

Some signs of stress are so subtle that they're easy to overlook. To evaluate the current level of stress in your life, read through the following list of statements and rate each one based on how it applies to you. Use the following scale: 0 for never true; 1 for rarely true; 2 for sometimes true; 3 for frequently true; 4 for always true.

Activities

_____ I completely lose interest in social activities and hobbies. The effort seems too great.

_____ I have a hard time knowing what I would like to do with free time. (For some suggestions, see 20 Instant Stress Relievers on page 220.)

_____ I tend to start more projects than I can possibly finish.

_____ I find myself feeling overwhelmed and out of control because there are too many demands on me. (Check out Simplify Your Life without Sacrifice on page 226.)

Self-Concept

_____ I feel that there is very little time for me in the day.

_____ I feel unappreciated by my family. (Be sure to read Be a Super Mom, Not Supermom on page 236.)

_____ I feel a sense of resentment and anger that I cannot really explain.

_____ I find that I often look for compliments and praise. (Don't miss When "Good Enough" Is Good Enough on page 230.)

Appetite

_____ I feel too tense or aggravated to eat.

_____ I crave coffee or cigarettes to keep me going.

_____ I need chocolate and/or other carbohydrates when I feel tired or down. (See Stop Feeding Your Emotions on page 170.)

_____ I often have cramps, nausea, or diarrhea.

Sleep

_____ I have trouble falling asleep. (For your best rest ever, see Help Yourself to More Sleep on page 93.)

_____ I do not feel rested even when I get a full night's sleep.

_____ I fall asleep earlier than I want to in the evening.

_____ I need a long nap in the afternoon.

Outlook

_____ I feel as though I've lost my sense of humor.

_____ I feel impatient and irritable.

_____ I am pessimistic about the future.

_____ I feel numb and emotionless.

_____ **Total**

Assessing Your Score

Once you have your total, find its place in the ranges below. In general, if your score is higher than 20, you'll definitely want to pay attention to the information and advice in the next five chapters. Aim to get your score into the low risk range.

_1 to 20._ You're at low risk for stress.

_21 to 40._ You run a mild risk for stress.

_41 to 60._ You're at moderate risk for stress. Try taking it easier.

_61 to 80._ You're in the high stress range. It's time to reprioritize.

31

Prescriptions for Total Serenity

"Honey, are you getting enough sleep?" your mother inquires over lunch, as your eyelids droop toward your salad.

"So, how long has it been?" your best friend asks about your soporific sex life.

"Looks like someone needs a vacation," your boss announces after reviewing your latest proposal.

As much as you resent their comments, deep down, you know that they're on to something. In your rush to handle all of your everyday obligations, important needs like love, laughter, sleep, and sex are being shuffled aside.

The problem is, these are the very things that should be women's top priorities, says Karen Rucker, M.D., chairman of the department of physical medicine and rehabilitation at Virginia Commonwealth University/Medical College of Virginia in Richmond. "Without them, everything else suffers," she explains. "Taking time for these things makes you not only happier but healthier as well."

That said, here are four "lifelong" prescriptions for your mind, body, and soul.

Laughter

Rx: At Least 30 Minutes per Day

You always knew that a good laugh could chase away the blues. But did you also know that laughing it up regularly with your friends and family can help

Feels Like You Never Left

A relaxing vacation can be the perfect salve for a stressed-out soul. But just how long can you expect those good vibrations to last?

Apparently, not as long as they should, according to a study at Tel Aviv University in Israel. Most of the 76 study participants reported fading good feelings within just three days of their return to reality. And within three weeks, their stress levels returned to pre-vacation status. Interestingly, women seemed able to sustain the afterglow longer than men.

What can you do to recapture that post-vacation mindset? For starters, identify some part of your vacation that you enjoyed and that you can incorporate into your daily routine. And make a point of taking relaxation breaks throughout the day—stretch at your desk or take a walk after dinner, for example.

fight off illnesses such as colds, flu, and even high blood pressure?

"Although laughter may not actually cure anything, it does boost immunity," says Kathleen Dillon, Ph.D., professor of psychology at Western New England College in Springfield, Massachusetts. Dr. Dillon discovered that breastfeeding mothers who laughed at their problems instead of spending time worrying about them had fewer incidences of colds and flu, as did their newborns.

Even watching two of your favorite TV sitcoms back to back may help you stay healthy. In a study at Loma Linda University School of Medicine in California, blood samples were taken from 10 students before, during, and after an hour-long comedy video. The samples showed that activated T cells, natural killer cells, and antibodies (the body's defense against viruses and infection) actually increased temporarily.

"You don't need 30 minutes of continuous belly laughter. A series of giggles and laughs throughout the day is just as good for you," says Clifford C. Kuhn, M.D., professor of psychiatry at the University of Louisville School of Medicine in Kentucky, who also teaches humor therapy.

So experiment. Try different types of media and collect your favorites, suggests Dr. Kuhn. Build yourself a home library of humorous books, videotapes, magazines, posters—anything that you can get your hands on to give yourself a chuckle whenever you need one. If you don't have the time for all that, just try to stop and savor those moments when you stumble onto something that you find absurd or silly, and then share your thoughts with a friend for a good laugh.

Love

Rx: Five Hugs per Day

"How much love we feel affects everything from our general well-being to how well our bodies can fight off disease," says Lillie Weiss, Ph.D., a psychologist in private practice in Phoenix. Researchers at Osijek University Hospital in Croatia found that among 137 volunteers, those who felt loved by family and friends had lower cholesterol levels than those who lacked emotional support. They also had healthier body mass indexes (BMIs)—an important indicator of heart disease risk—than those who felt unfulfilled in relationships with others.

Try to give or receive five hugs a day. If there's no one around, give yourself one. "Loving yourself is the first step toward getting more love in your life," says Dr. Weiss. "Also consider getting a pet. Animals give unconditional love."

Finally, start showing love to others, says Dr. Weiss. Invite someone out to lunch. Call people you haven't spoken to in a while. "The good feelings you give will eventually come back to you," she says.

Sleep

Rx: Eight Hours per Day

Most of us wouldn't dream of driving when we know we've had a few too many. Yet every day, millions of us get behind the wheel after having too little sleep—a practice, studies show, that can be more dangerous than driving drunk.

Why aren't we getting enough sleep? One reason is that "society regards the act of 'sleeping in' as wasteful," says Mark R. Pressman, Ph.D., associate director of the sleep disorders center at Lankenau Hospital in Wynnewood, Pennsylvania. "Many of us feel pressured to stay up later and get up earlier in order to get more done."

Women tend to be more sleep-deprived than men because of overwhelming family and work responsibilities. Scrimping on sleep isn't healthy, since a single night of deprivation can significantly weaken your immune system.

Although sleep requirements vary from person to person, most of us end up functioning best with roughly eight hours of shut-eye a night. So how can you tell how much sleep is right for you? "You'll know you're getting enough if you wake up some mornings without using your alarm clock," says Lynne Lamberg, author of *Body Rhythms: Chronobiology and Peak Performance*.

If you know that your body needs more sleep, but you don't know how much, try sneaking into bed just 15 minutes earlier each evening. If your usual bedtime is midnight, for example, get under the covers at 11:45 one night,

11:30 the next, and so on until you begin waking up naturally before your alarm goes off. That's your ideal schedule.

Once you're back on track, here's how to ensure that you continue to get enough sleep: If you smoke, quit; exercise regularly (aim for at least three workouts a week); and go to bed and wake up at about the same times every day—including weekends and days off.

Sexual Contact

Rx: At Least Once per Day

For married couples, great sex is like a weekend getaway. It's so wonderful, you wonder why you don't do it more often, and you vow to "return" soon. Then life gets in the way, and sex ends up on a shelf along with a huge stack of bed-and-breakfast brochures.

"Most people say that if it weren't for their children, their hectic schedules, and their jobs, they'd be having a lot more sex," says Bernie Zilbergeld, Ph.D., a sex therapist in Oakland, California, and author of *The New Male Sexuality*. "Most men and women—married or single—are not satisfied with how much sex they're getting." This isn't healthy, especially since experts believe that sex is more important than many of the other "priorities" that push it aside.

"There are very few things that make you feel as good about yourself as sex does," says Dr. Zilbergeld. "It also helps give you a better night's sleep and provides moderate exercise."

Some women find that sexual activity is also a great stress reliever, says Tara Roth Madden, author of *Romance on the Run: Five Minutes of Quality Sex for Busy Couples*. That's because orgasmic waves are fueled by natural brain chemicals known as endorphins, the same ones that give runners a mood-elevating "high" after a good workout. It's these chemicals that create a state of bliss after sex as well.

Everyone's sexual needs are different, so you shouldn't insist on having sex with your mate a set number times a week, says Dr. Zilbergeld. Instead, make a point to have some sort of sexual contact with your partner at least once a day, whether it's a passionate good-morning kiss, touching each other in the evening, or leaving a sexy phone message during the day. Also try to take care of your body. Regular exercise boosts your metabolic rate and hormone levels, which not only puts you in the mood more often but also gives you extra energy for quality time between the sheets.

Finally, never dismiss the power of the quickie, Madden says. "Try intentionally giving limited time to each other," she advises. "You'll be amazed how a few short sexual encounters can charge your sex life."

32

20 Instant Stress Relievers

Fact of life number one: When you least expect it, you're going to get hit with one hair-pulling, nail-biting, crazy-making thing or another—a flat tire, a bounced check, a kid's less-than-stellar report card. Fact of life number two: There is no limit to the number of such things that can hit you in a day.

"Women are probably under more stress than ever before," says Camille Lloyd, Ph.D., professor in the department of psychiatry and behavioral sciences at the University of Texas Medical School at Houston. And that's not healthy. Studies suggest that your body's physical reaction to high levels of sustained stress—increased blood pressure, an outpouring of adrenaline, and other changes—makes you more susceptible to heart disease and other serious health problems.

On a day-to-day basis, stress may leave you feeling depressed, irritable, despairing, or edgy, says Sharon Greenburg, Ph.D., a clinical psychologist in private practice in Chicago. You may find that you can't sleep, concentrate, or recall things. You may get headaches.

On-the-Spot Calm

Because stress can be so destructive to your physical and emotional health, you want to do whatever you can to defuse it. These expert-approved tactics can help.

Do Guys Have More to Be Happy About?

Scientists have long known that women are more likely than men to experience depression, but they could never quite explain why. New research suggests that it may have something to do with serotonin, a chemical involved in the transmission of mood messages within the brain.

In a small preliminary study conducted at McGill University in Montreal, researchers found that men produce 52 percent more serotonin than women. This is one of the most significant differences between the brains of men and women that is not related to hormones, the researchers concluded.

These findings may someday help doctors understand why more women suffer from depression, notes Simon N. Young, Ph.D., professor in the department of psychiatry, division of neurochemistry, at McGill University. He says the next step will be to look at men and women with specific conditions that are affected by serotonin levels.

Studies like this one may also prompt greater interest in examining the connection between hormones and serotonin. Specifically, researchers may one day look into how oral contraceptives and hormone replacement therapy influence serotonin levels, says David H. Schwartz, Ph.D., a neuroscientist who is tracking serotonin research for the Weinberg Group, a scientific consulting organization in New York City.

Whether the new information about serotonin will change the way depression is treated in either sex is anyone's guess. "One day, data like this may affect the kinds of medications prescribed for depression," says Dr. Schwartz. For example, selective serotonin drugs may prove to be a more effective choice for women than other types of medications.

Work it off. The next time stress gives you the urge to curl into the fetal position, take a quick walk or jog instead. A study conducted at the University of Illinois at Urbana–Champaign found that exercise relaxes you more than if you just sat around being a slug. The study monitored 34 moderately active students in three different environments: sitting quietly in a room, jogging at their own pace in a laboratory, and working out wherever they liked. Those who sat on their duffs weren't any more relaxed after 20 minutes, but those who worked out experienced a 20 percent reduction in their anxiety levels, reports Edward McAuley, Ph.D., professor of kinesiology at the university.

Touch your toes. No, not that way. Give your feet a gentle massage. Concentrating on your troubled soles will get your mind off your troubled soul. First, press your thumbs into your arches, then do the same over every square inch of your soles. Finally, move each toe from side to side and from front to back.

Have a ball. Chinese exercise balls are steeped in tradition and mystery. First made during the Ming Dynasty, Baoding Iron Balls (from Baoding, China) contain a sounding plate that emits a low, soothing ring when you roll them in the palm of your hand. According to traditional Chinese medical theory, the manipulation of these spheres is a form of self-acupressure, which benefits the entire body.

Here's how to handle the balls: Take both of them in one hand and roll them in a circle, clockwise or counterclockwise, from finger to finger in sequence. The balls should revolve around each other in a smooth, continuous motion. Alternate hands.

Stretch out. To relax your muscles from head to toe, do a full-body stretch while lying face-up on an exercise mat. Start with your feet: Tense them and curl your toes for 10 seconds, then release. Continue up your body, tensing and relaxing your thighs, buttocks, abdominal muscles, back, shoulders, arms, hands, neck, and face. When you finish, your entire body should feel loose, and your mind should be calm.

Take time for tea. Decaffeinated tea, that is. The caffeine in regular tea gives you a boost that's followed by an even bigger slump. On the other hand, some decaf teas contain herbs that actually calm jangled nerves. "Sipping a cup of herbal tea nourishes your nerves, soothes you with its warmth, and relaxes you with its sweet fragrance," says Brigitte Mars, an herbalist in Boulder, Colorado. Two tasty teas for sipping away stress: Lipton Soothing Moments Herbal Tea in Gentle Orange and Lemon Soother flavors.

Get steamed. Relaxing your facial muscles can give your spirits a lift. And one of the easiest ways to do it is with a facial steaming. In a large bowl, steep three bags of chamomile tea in a half-quart of boiling water. Sit with your face over the bowl, no less than 12 inches from the water. Tent a towel over your head to trap the steam. If your face gets too hot, lift a corner of the towel to vent some of the steam. Keep your eyes closed and breathe deeply for about 10 minutes.

Go for a soak. Everyone has heard that lounging in a steaming tub soothes jangled nerves. But do you know how hot the water should be? About the same temperature as your skin—between 90° and 95°F, recommends Jens Henriksen, M.D., a rheumatologist and pain management specialist in Rushville, Georgia.

Turn your eyes skyward. Head for the hills. Or the beach. Or an open field. "Watching the clouds roll by is a form of meditation," says Aaron Katcher, M.D., a psychiatrist in Wayne, Pennsylvania. By focusing on nature, you turn your thoughts away from your worries.

Take a deep breath. Focusing on your inhalations and exhalations can produce a sense of calm and balance in your body, points out Janet R. Messer, Ph.D., a psychologist in Eugene, Oregon. Even better, you can do it anytime, anywhere—standing, sitting, or lying down. Begin by closing your eyes; make sure your back is straight. Slowly inhale through your nose, feeling your lungs fill from bottom to top. Then exhale through your nose, emptying your lungs from top to bottom. Focus your attention on a spot at the center of your belly, about an inch below your navel. As you inhale, feel your diaphragm being pulled down toward this point. Continue this breathing exercise until you feel relaxed.

Put pen to paper. Writing about your frustrations allows you to vent without having to reveal your feelings to someone else, psychologists say. Every evening, take a few minutes to scribble down anything that may be troubling you. Be honest. Don't worry about grammar, and don't censor your words. This exercise is intended to help you work through your feelings, not craft the great American novel. Above all else, don't show your journal to anyone.

Throw the book at stress. Reading provides a great escape from the real world. But be careful when choosing a book to snuggle up with. If you devour tomes about work issues, you may actually boost your stress level, especially if your job is a source of tension. Indulge in a purely fun read.

Color away the blues. The next time stress strikes, dive into that familiar green and yellow box and grab a crayon. Adult colorers are more common than you might think, according to Binney and Smith, the Easton, Pennsylvania–based maker of Crayola products. Why? Coloring is fun and instantly rewarding, it lowers blood pressure, and it's relaxing. And for folks who are into aromatherapy, Crayola Magic Scent crayons come in stress-busting aromas, including leather jacket, lumber, lilac, shampoo, and new car.

Root, root, root for the home team. Take in a game of the sport of your choice. Yelling at the umpire or referee is a great way to release pent-up anger and frustration. "By being part of an audience, you can express hostility in a nondestructive manner," says Roger Thies, Ph.D., associate professor of physiology at the University of Oklahoma Health Sciences Center in Oklahoma City. And if your team wins, your spirits rise even more. "We identify with the players," he explains. "When they triumph, we triumph with them."

Head for the mall. Take a leisurely stroll through one of the many stores stocked with scented soaps, lotions, and other sensuous indulgences. Savor the aroma of scented hand cream, the casual chatter of friendly salesclerks, the lift you feel when you purchase that special facial scrub. "As the saying goes, 'When the going gets tough, the tough go shopping,'" says Billie Scott of Simon Property Group, operators of Mall of America, the most visited mall in the United States. But if your budget is tight, don't feel obligated to buy. Just window-shopping or power-walking around the mall will boost your mood.

Burst your bubble. In one study, students reduced tension by popping bubble-wrap packing material. How does it work? "Bubble popping relaxes your muscles," explains Kathleen Dillon, Ph.D., professor of psychology at Western New England College in Springfield, Massachusetts, and the study's author. The bigger the bubble, the better the stress reduction. To pack up your troubles, pick up some wrap. If you don't have any lying around the office, check your nearest office supply store.

Postpone picking up. If you're expecting a stressful phone call, don't dive for the receiver on the first ring. Wait two or three rings, then pick up. Not responding immediately can help defuse stress, says Ronald Nathan, Ph.D., professor of family practice and psychiatry at Albany Medical College in New York. As the phone rings, breathe deeply. As you exhale, imagine your body becoming limp, like a rag doll's. Taking your time will give you a feeling of control, Dr. Nathan explains. And that control will make you feel calmer and competent to handle the crisis.

Make time fly. Ditch your watch after work. You'll be better able to relax and enjoy your free hours.

Just don't do it. Look at your life. Are you taking on too much? If you're organizing your church's annual picnic, leading a scout troop, bowling one night a week, and—oh, yeah—running a family and pursuing a career, you have to learn to say no to something. "Prune your activity branches," suggests Richard Swenson, M.D., author of *Margin: Restoring Emotional, Physical, Financial, and Time Reserves to Overloaded Lives*.

Put things in perspective. Differentiate between the stressors you can change and those you can't, advises Denis Waitley, a motivational/educational speaker based in Rancho Santa Fe, California. His strategy for defusing stress: First, list all of the personal and work issues that create stress for you. Then highlight the items you can control and transfer them to a separate list. For example, if your desk is a mess, you can clean it up.

Next, look at the stressors you think you can't control. Maybe you just need a creative way to take charge of them. For example, if you hate photocopying, ask your supervisor if you can delegate the task.

What about the stressors you can't eliminate? Make the best of them. You can't change stressors such as bad weather and inflation, but you can stop the stress that comes from dwelling on them. The Serenity Prayer says it best: Try to accept the things you can't change; find the courage to change the things you can; and have the wisdom to know the difference.

Call for help. People are usually willing to help someone in need, says Morton Hunt, author of *The Compassionate Beast: What Science Is Discovering about the Humane Side of Humankind*. So if you're feeling alone and abandoned, it's probably not because people don't care. It's more likely because you're not being clear about what you need. Ask precisely and directly. And don't forget to say thank you.

33 Simplify Your Life without Sacrifice

You've picked your closets clean. You've trimmed your magazine subscriptions to what you have time to read—not one page more. With tricks for doing just about everything faster, from mowing the lawn to bundling the kids off to school, you tear through your calendar like that Looney Tunes creation known as the Tasmanian Devil.

So why, at the end of each day, do you feel as though someone has dropped an anvil on your head?

Simplifying your life is all well and good. But too often you rush to save time, only to end up filling it with another task. What you really want to do is not just cut corners or speed up a process but streamline your life as well. That way, you'll have "real time" each day to curl up with a good book, slip away for an after-dinner stroll, or just do nothing (for a change).

Making Changes Painlessly

The following tips are designed to truly make your life simpler. The folks who've provided this advice aren't your run-of-the-mill, jargon-spouting experts. And they're not the Oprahs and the Madonnas of the world who have entire staffs to simplify their lives for them. These are real people who really are doing it all. Among them is a mother of quintuplets, the president of a

Where Does the Time Go?

Americans are overworked, stressed out, and desperate for a few hours to themselves, right? Not necessarily. Research has shown that Americans have more free time than ever. The problem is how we use it.

In analyzing the daily diaries of 10,000 Americans over a 20-year period, Geoffrey Godbey, Ph.D., and John P. Robinson, Ph.D., co-authors of *Time for Life*, found that the average person has gained five hours of free time per week. A review of data from 1995 shows that the trend is continuing. So why do we feel harried?

"Our extra time comes in small bursts scattered through the workweek," explains Dr. Godbey, professor of leisure studies at Pennsylvania State University in University Park. "People come home a little earlier, but work is seeping into their weekends. What people want is large chunks of time, so they can make a garden or coach a softball team."

Time devoted to such activities has fallen. Instead, we fill our snippets of freedom with sitcoms. Of the 40 hours of free time we have every week, we spend 16 hours watching TV. And the adults who watch the most TV are the least likely to socialize with friends, take classes, or play sports.

So here's an easy way to find leisure time: Turn off the tube. There—you're 16 hours richer.

HEALTH FLASH

---

major university, and a rat-race dropout sailing around the world—solo. Each of them adds a unique twist to the word *simplify*.

So before you decide that your life is muddled beyond hope, read on. You'll see for yourself that simplifying can indeed be simple.

Cancel the paper. Most major newspapers (and many smaller ones) are on the Web, and going there is more efficient all around. Consider:

❖ News online is usually fresher than the version on your doorstep.
❖ In all but a handful of cases, online newspapers are free (no bills to pay).
❖ There's no need to stop delivery when you're on vacation—or to drive a month's worth of papers to the recycling center.
❖ You don't waste time scrubbing ink off your hands.

Pass the bills. Want to save paper, stamps, and licking time? Many major utilities, insurance companies, and lenders can automatically tap your bank account whenever a bill is due. Contact your bank to find out how.

Lose your answering machine. Bid farewell to call-waiting and junk those tiny cassettes that fill up your drawers and seem to jam on all but the most banal of messages. How can you do that? With residential voice mail. Just like at work, you can take messages whether you're on the other line or away from home—or simply not in the mood to chat. Plus, you can send messages without having to talk to a real live person (provided that person has voice mail, too). Ask your phone company for details.

Buy a notebook and keep it handy. Jotting down shopping lists and plot lines for your Great American Novel is a good idea. Just don't do it on whatever scrap happens to be lying around. Merge such imperatives onto one master list. And make it big, so it's easy to find.

Phone ahead. Right before you leave for your appointment with the dentist, optometrist, or whatever "-ist" you're due to see, call to make sure the good doctor is running on schedule. You have better things to do with your time than to sit around listening to Muzak.

Make them come to you. Hunt around for a dry-cleaning service that picks up and delivers. If you're a regular, you just might merit special treatment.

Hire a haggler. Shopping for a new car can feel like a boxing match. So get someone to step in the ring for you. A service called CarSource will contact dealerships within a 60- to 90-mile radius of your home to find the very best deal on the make and model you're looking for. All you have to do is go to the dealership to inspect your new vehicle and hand over the check. The fee runs from $275 to $675, depending on the price of the car—but CarSource guarantees savings from $1,000 to $12,000.

For more information, call CarSource directly. The 800 number is available from toll-free directory assistance.

Take that string off your finger. It's tough to live simply when your brain is constantly buzzing in remember mode: "What am I forgetting today? Did I write it down? And where is my datebook, anyway?" Banish these worries with a single pen stroke—in your checkbook. For a one-time fee, a Denver outfit called Never Forget Again will see to it that Aunt Verna's birthday never again slips by unnoticed. (You'll receive a postcard one week before each event you list.) You can obtain the company's 800 number by calling toll-free directory assistance.

Stamp out stress. If you have a credit card, cross the post office off your to-do list and pick up the phone. The U.S. Postal Service will deliver stamps to your mailbox within approximately five business days. One caveat: You must place a minimum order of 45 stamps.

Get to know your librarian. Even if your local library doesn't have a cappuccino bar, it still beats out the local Book-Mart. Why? Look no further than the teetering pile of "must-reads" on your nightstand. Buy a book, and its presence is a nagging reminder of unfinished business until you've read every last chapter. And then it lies around your house for another 10 years. Borrow a book from the library, and you can simply dump it in the night-return box and be free of it.

Do your work—and no one else's. The fastest way to add to your workload is to gain a reputation as a know-it-all. "A man I know liked to be thought of as the resident expert, so whenever there was a problem, he was the guy to turn to," says C. Steven Manley, Ph.D., a psychologist in Dallas. "He ended up working until midnight just to finish his own work."

Close the book. "Read any good books lately?" Good luck trying to escape a dinner party without hearing that one. Thing is, staying hip to the latest best-sellers can be draining, to say the least. Instead, simply read the reviews (the *New York Times Book Review* is a sure bet). They dish up enough highlights to see you through any casual conversation, and they provide ready-made commentary to boot. Before long, you'll be spouting phrases like "spellbinding narrative" without even trying.

Map things out. Nothing turns a road trip upside down more quickly than a missed exit or mangled directions. Bypass these snafus by checking the Internet for Web sites that provide mapping services. Simply type in your starting point and your destination. Within seconds, you'll get directions so detailed that they'll knock your socks off.

34

When "Good Enough" Is Good Enough

Perfectionism has its place. For Olympic gymnasts, it can mean the difference between the gold and silver medals. For accountants, it can mean the difference between a client getting a tax refund and owing the IRS money. For circus knife-throwers . . . well, you get the idea.

When it means being accurate and thorough, perfectionism is certainly an admirable quality. But when it runs amok—when you set unrealistic standards for yourself, for example, or you consider anything less than perfect unacceptable—it can be surprisingly detrimental to your personal and professional lives.

Gone Too Far

"Perfectionism is an important trait to have in order to get ahead in life, to achieve and accomplish," says Allan Mallinger, M.D., a San Diego psychiatrist and author of *Too Perfect: When Being in Control Gets Out of Control*. "But when it becomes rigid and driven, when it doesn't ebb and flow, it can be too much of a good thing. Excessive thoroughness means that it can take forever to get something done."

On the continuum of what mental health professionals call obsessive/compulsive behavior (which at its worst can manifest itself as an anxiety disorder), perfectionism is at the low end. But the slope gets slippery with the increasing need for control. Men and women are equally likely to be perfectionists. Experts say, however, that women who work in mostly male offices may be prone to perfectionism if they are overly concerned about trying to prove their worth. "They're afraid someone is going to criticize them," says Marilyn Moats Kennedy, career counselor and author of the monthly newsletter *Kennedy's Career Strategist.* "It's a form of insecurity."

The irony, adds Dr. Mallinger, is that despite all of the attention perfectionists pay to their work, they don't even enjoy the results. "Even when they do their jobs well, they're immediately focusing on what they've done wrong and how they could have done better," he says. Other projects languish while the perfectionist struggles over every detail of the task at hand. Because of their need for control, perfectionists may also have trouble making decisions and commitments, delegating, and taking risks. And that, says Dr. Mallinger, can mean lost opportunities for growth and fulfillment.

In Search of Respect

Why does a person become a perfectionist? Often she's striving to earn someone else's approval. The irony is that she probably doesn't realize it, even when those around her do.

Are You Too Perfect?

The pursuit of perfectionism can cause unnecessary stress, destroy relationships, and otherwise wreak havoc on your personal and professional lives. The following quiz can help you determine whether your perfectionist streak may be working against you. Circle the letter of the statement that most applies to you.

1. You ask your assistant to pull together some figures for an upcoming budget meeting. A week later, she hasn't even started. You:
   A. Do it yourself—it was probably too complicated for her to handle anyway
   B. Let her take her time—you have more important tasks that need your attention
   C. Firmly remind her that you need the job done now—and done right

2. A co-worker compliments you on the new suit that you're wearing. You assume that she:
   A. Admires your sense of style
   B. Thinks you usually look like a slob
   C. Is trying to find out where you're interviewing for another job

3. Your boss asks you to make a presentation to the entire staff next month, but you're terrified by the thought of speaking in public. You:
   A. Promise your boss that you'll do a great job and enroll in the first public speaking class you can find
   B. Promise your boss that you'll do a great job, then spend the rest of the day re-alphabetizing your Rolodex
   C. Tell your boss thanks but no thanks and let the chips fall where they may

4. There's no getting out of it. You have to make that presentation. Which task do you tackle first?
   A. The research—if you're going to get up there, you'd better know everything there is to know about the subject

Most perfectionists learn their behavior from a boss or a parent, and they fear punishment if they make mistakes. "Often they were raised in families where whatever they did wasn't good enough," says J. Clayton Lafferty, Ph.D., psychologist at Human Synergistics International, a management consulting firm in Plymouth, Michigan. "So they turned to perfectionism, putting incredible demands on themselves and projecting those demands onto others."

In today's volatile workplace, where rampant downsizing translates to more work for everyone, being a perfectionist can be career suicide. "People who are

B. The report—all of the higher-ups are going to be reading what you write, so it needs to be solid

C. The seating plan—you don't want your boss (or her boss, for that matter) to be stuck next to the office kook

5. Congratulations! You're getting promoted, and you're going to hand-pick your replacement You:

A. Put an ad in the paper and hire the first decent person to respond; after all, you have more important things to do now

B. Put an ad in the paper, interview dozens of qualified people, ask every competent person you know for input, and never hire anyone

C. Put an ad in the paper, interview dozens of qualified people, ask them to do a sample project, re-interview the top candidates, and hire the one who impresses you most

6. Your work involves:

A. Information—programming, accounting, research

B. People—sales, teaching, medicine

C. Creativity—photography, advertising, writing

Answers

1. Give yourself one point If you chose A. Perfectionists hate delegating even menial tasks.
2. One point for B or C. To a perfectionist, a compliment always has a hidden meaning.
3. One point for B. Perfectionists are notorious procrastinators.
4. One point for C. Because of their fear of failure, perfectionists tend to focus on the little, meaningless tasks instead of the big picture.
5. One point for B. Perfectionists are tortured by making decisions.
6. One point for A, B, or C. You'd think perfectionists would be number crunchers, but they have all kinds of jobs.

Count up your points. If you have four or more, perfectionism may be a problem for you.

being asked to do too much aren't going to be able to do everything perfectly," says Dr. Mallinger. "But perfectionists can't handle that. They have trouble sleeping, they get irritable, and they have interpersonal problems at work—all because they can't adapt to the new requirements of this economy."

An obsession with perfection can be especially counterproductive at managerial and executive levels. "Very few organizations have key people who are perfectionistic, because they're too dogmatic," says Dr. Lafferty. "Companies simply can't afford them."

One of Dr. Lafferty's clients was a young executive who had a bright future in publishing. "But she was about to lose her job because no one could stand her," he recalls. "She second-guessed every decision anyone made and always zeroed in on the flaws rather than the strengths in her colleagues' work. She was responsible for tremendous turnover because people just left. And she fired more talent than she herself had. Her bosses told her she had to change or she would be fired."

Perfectionists are also reluctant to admit their own fallibility, which can be dangerous in environments where mistakes must be admitted so that disaster can be avoided. In fact, one study found that many airplane accidents can be attributed to the pilots' perfectionism. Their unwillingness to admit—and thus correct—crucial errors led to needless tragedy.

And if perfectionism infects the entire corporate culture, the results can be disastrous. Dr. Lafferty cites at least one major company that nearly caused its own collapse by setting sales goals so high that it was never able to meet them.

Making Yourself Sick

Maintaining a superhuman image can exact a high price outside the office as well as within it. In Dr. Lafferty's 10-year study of managers and professionals, people whom he identified as perfectionists (based on their descriptions of themselves) had a high frequency not only of diminished job performance but also of illness.

Considering the pressure that perfectionists put on themselves, the fact that they have a greater tendency toward stress-related illness—from headaches to gastrointestinal problems to chest pains—comes as no surprise. They are also prone to depression and even suicide because they are so afraid of failure.

If a perfectionist can't live up to her own expectations, chances are that no one in her life can either. Marriage between a perfectionist and a nonperfectionist can be an absolute nightmare. "Even the children become alienated," says Dr. Lafferty. "If they could leave home at five years old, they probably would."

The Warning Signs

How do you know if you're being a perfectionist? "When you're missing deadlines, when you consistently go down to the wire on a project, when you struggle to make sure it's perfect," says Kennedy. "The truth is that you're doing it not for the sake of the job or because it needs to be done but because it makes *you* feel better."

If you suspect that your perfectionism is holding you back, Dr. Lafferty recommends that you first confront the problem with the help of a therapist. You need to admit to yourself that you're not as effective as you think you are, though coming to terms with your own faults won't be easy. "They almost always come as a great surprise," says Dr. Lafferty.

The next step is to get feedback from your co-workers, subordinates, and family—if you can bear it. "People will tell you the truth about your behavior," says Dr. Lafferty. "Promise not to disagree with what they say."

Ask them questions, such as what your behavior has cost you in terms of your relationships with them. "You have to recognize what the price has been," says Dr. Mallinger. "That's the leverage that's going to make you change."

Letting Go

Once you've come to terms with your unhealthy attitude, you can concentrate on changing your habits. At work, refocus your energy on achievement, on getting the job done. Write down how much time you spend on everything you do, from phone calls to big projects. That way, you can see where your hours go. "Ask yourself whether the time is productive—because time is indeed money—or whether you're simply gilding the lily," advises Kennedy.

Don't let minor tasks eat up your attention, and don't get mired in details. Delegate where possible—you can't do everything yourself. Allow yourself to let something be imperfect, especially a less important project. Remind yourself, "I have more important things to do." It's a statement about your own value, recognizing that this is all you can give right now.

And don't be afraid to laugh at yourself when you feel yourself giving in to perfectionism. "Take a framed picture that's hanging on a wall and set it askew," suggests Nicole, a teacher in Baltimore. "Then test yourself to see how long you'll let it stay that way. When I realized that I couldn't let it be, I also realized how crazy I was."

There's no panacea for perfectionism, admits Dr. Lafferty. "A perfectionist is like a magnificent computer with molasses poured into its keyboard," he says. "The solution isn't to redesign the computer but to get the molasses out of the keyboard."

Remember that practice may indeed make perfect. But "perfect" isn't all that it's cracked up to be.

Be a Super Mom, Not Supermom

Becoming a mother often means making sacrifices for the sake of the children. Certainly, it's a noble gesture. But when does it go too far?

In the following excerpt from her book The Sacrificial Mother: Escaping the Trap of Self-Denial, *author Carin Rubenstein, Ph.D., explores why women instinctively give up so much for their families—and how they can keep from losing sight of themselves.*

I'd like to tell you about my pickle revelation.

In my family, we all love pickles—just about any kind of pickle. But if there's only one pickle left, if it's the last pickle in the jar, I always give it to my children. They each get half a pickle, and I get none. This is how it has always been and, I imagine, how it will always be.

My husband laughs about this, about my willingness to give up the last pickle in the jar. "I would never do that," he says. It's true. Faced with the last pickle, he simply eats it and recycles the jar. It does not occur to him to deny himself a pickle for his children. "That's a mom thing," he says. Thinking about it, I realize that many mothers I know would, in fact, give up the last pickle for their children.

Mothers deny themselves for their children just about every day. Some sacrifice by staying home all day when they'd really rather go to work. Others sacrifice by going to work when they yearn to be at home. Whatever their situation, many mothers sacrifice naturally, automatically, and without question. They sacrifice not just for their obviously needy newborns but for their rambunctious toddlers and inquisitive six-year-olds, for their newly independent fifth-graders and their moody teenagers. Examples of the ways in which women sacrifice for their children are humdrum, unexceptional, expected.

Do You Fit the Mold?

For many women, true sacrifice goes far deeper than the above examples. It means always thinking of their children's needs first. It means feeling guilty for not always being the most giving, most supportive, most caring mother. It means making sacrifice a way of life.

Here, in no particular order, are some signs that you may be a sacrificial mother.

- You spend at least one-third of your day thinking about something your child needs or wants or agonizing about what you should have done or wish you had done for your child.
- You can't remember the last time you spent more than one hour by yourself.
- You and your spouse have not had an evening out by yourselves since your last anniversary.
- When your daughter is devastated by something someone said to her at school, so are you.
- When your son forgets his lunch box at home, you drop it off at his school before noon, even if it is the third time this month. Working mother corollary: If you can't take his lunch because you're at work, you feel guilty about it all day.
- You'd rather buy your children new overalls than get yourself a new pair of jeans.
- If you go away for several days, you tape-record yourself reading stories to your children. Or you leave little notes. Or you shower them with presents when you return.
- Your children don't know how to turn on the washing machine or how to fold socks. (This applies to any child over age 8.)

My research has shown that about 8 of 10 mothers often sacrifice their own needs and desires for their children. And nearly as many believe that this sacrifice is their duty as a mother. They sacrifice so much and so often because they feel certain their sacrifices will ultimately benefit their children. But it's possible that mothers who sacrifice too much harm both themselves and their children in the process.

Too Much of a Good Thing

One of the most obvious consequences of sacrifice is a simple and overwhelming loss of sense of self and self-esteem. This cyclone of sacrifice leaves a trail of emotional debris that includes personal vulnerability, emotional instability, and physical illness. I think many mothers sense that too much sacrifice isn't healthy. But they do it anyway, hoping and praying that if they sacrifice enough, they will be transformed into that enviable and elusive object of desire: the perfect wife and mother. Sadly, though, they're mistaken. When I ask them to rate themselves, sacrificial mothers say they fail at being the best possible wife and lover and mother.

At my sacrificial peak, I never gave myself a thought. I felt I simply didn't matter. I was in such bad shape that I didn't bother to figure out what I thought about anything. I'd start an argument with my husband but be unable to articulate why he was wrong and I was right. I'd show up to vote in a local election and discover that I didn't have an opinion either way. I was sleepwalking through my life for what I thought was the sake of my children.

This personal vanishing act happens to many mothers who sacrifice too much. They lose their ability to care about and for themselves, and it's one of the reasons why their self-esteem plummets so precipitously. With this lack of self-respect comes a creeping self-doubt, a suspicion that nothing you do or say is all that important.

When I compare mothers' opinions of their looks with how childless women see themselves, I find that mothers are less happy with their physical appearance. And sacrificial mothers are the most distressed of all, in part because they rarely take time to make any improvements. Sacrificial mothers focus on their children with such ferocity and resolve that they have little time or energy to pay attention to their image.

The Costs of Sacrifice

The psychological troubles associated with being sacrificial add up to a mountain of melancholy. Compared with other women, twice as many sacrificial mothers have psychological problems. Twice as many of them feel irritable, have trouble sleeping, and have difficulty concentrating. Twice as many feel guilty and terribly lonely. They have more headaches, stomach problems, and muscle aches. They feel less successful in life than other mothers, and they're much more unhappy with their friendships, their work, and the way their lives are going.

Sacrificial mothers are also angrier than other women. And mothers in general are angrier than fathers. While parenthood is difficult for both partners, it's most distressing and painful for mothers because it costs them more socially and emotionally. When sociologists Catherine Ross, Ph.D., and Marieke Van Willigen, Ph.D., of Ohio State University in Columbus, studied a random group of adults, they found that women were angrier than men and that each additional child cranked up the mothers' anger levels even higher.

Part of what makes a sacrificial mother so angry is that she gives and gives and gives to the point where she feels trapped by the "should-bes"—all of the things she should be doing for her children and other family members. Yet she forgets what is equally important: all of the things she should be doing for herself.

It's no surprise, then, that her sensuality seems to disappear from the face of the earth. Many sacrificial mothers completely lose interest in anything sexual. Their warped logic goes like this: "If it feels good, I don 't deserve it, so I won't do it—and you can't make me." On top of all of this, they're almost too tired to breathe, let alone to think sexy thoughts.

Sexual frustration runs high among sacrificial mothers. Compared with other mothers, they feel less successful as lovers, and they're less satisfied with their sex lives. Fewer of them say they're in passionate love with their husbands. It's as if all of the sexual fervor and lust have been sucked out and those energies redirected to their children.

Sacrifice is also bad for a woman's physical health. I'm no longer amazed when moms whisper confessions to me about headaches and allergies, stomach pains and backaches, colds and fevers. Sacrificial mothers have more physical symptoms than other women and men. They also visit their doctors more often—at least five times a year.

Raising Kids That Are Out of Control

The driving force behind all of this sacrifice is the belief that our children will be better off because of it. Of course, good parenting does require some sacrifices. But why should Mom make all of them? And why do we believe that more is better? The truth is that too much sacrifice can actually harm children.

By sacrificing too much, a mother fosters dependency in her children. By always putting her children's needs first, a sacrificial mother leads them to believe that they have a right to rule the family and everyone in it. They feel princely because Mom feels servile.

Over the years, children with a sacrificial mother learn not to respect her. Because she allows herself to be treated like the household bath mat, that's how they come to view her. You can hear the lack of respect, the mix of disdain and impatience, in the way children of a sacrificial mother speak to her—as if she were too slow or ignorant to understand what they're saying.

It's a telling sign that a mother is sacrificial if her children are often rude, nasty, and ungrateful. On a visit to a party store, I listened as a six-year-old berated his mother for her ignorance of cartoon heroes, while she was trying to choose the most perfect plates and napkins for his birthday celebration.

Be Good to Yourself

You know that you can't throw your kids into a closet with some healthful snacks and a television set, lock the door, and get on with your life. Taking good care of babies and children always requires an enormous amount of selflessness and devotion. And sacrifice is not a matter of choice, despite the fact that it doesn't always help mothers or their children. Because sacrifice may be the result of some female biological urge, it can't—and shouldn't—be eradicated. But this doesn't mean that mothers live to be the only ones who sacrifice all the time, the only ones who discount themselves for the sake of the children.

Women have to learn to let go of some of the sacrifice and to grab hold of self. I call this talent selfism, or the art of learning to be a selfist.

To be able to care for others well, a woman needs to be able to love herself. To give to others, she has to learn how to take for herself. If mothers could only show themselves a fraction of the affection and attention they give to their children, they would be so much better off. They need to reserve some emotional energy for themselves, some room for their own needs and desires and dreams.

Being a selfist is not at all the same as being selfish. A selfist mother is one who can devote herself both to her children and to herself. She respects her children's wishes as well as her own. She can think of children first without thinking of children only. She can love her children with wild abandon and joy. But as a selfist, she makes a point of being good to herself by coddling herself when she's sick, setting aside time to read books and magazines that she likes, and saving money to be able to get her hair cut or to have coffee with friends. She knows that to function as a wife and a mother and a decent human being, she needs to recharge her own batteries nearly every day.

When I compare selfist mothers with others, the differences between the two groups are striking and dramatic. Selfist mothers are happier with just about every aspect of their lives—their marriages, their work, their intellectual abilities, their friends, their bodies, the way they look, and how their lives are going. Because they're able to treat themselves well, they have an optimistic outlook about everything that counts. They feel in charge; they feel competent.

Selfist mothers are less likely to feel depressed or angry. They also have a greater capacity to express their emotions. They avoid becoming emotionally constipated because they're never blocked by the unspoken resentment and frustrations that trouble so many sacrificial mothers.

It shouldn't come as too much of a surprise, then, that selfist mothers also have higher self-esteem and greater self-confidence. They even think of themselves as being more intelligent and more attractive than other mothers do. They like themselves more, so they treat themselves better. And the better they treat themselves, the more pride they feel. It's a self-fulfilling prophecy, one that enables selfist women to deal with the world on their own terms.

Four Steps to Selfism

Most sacrificial mothers have no idea how to go about behaving or feeling like selfists. My plan for achieving self-love does not preclude sacrifice, because children will always need an adult who is willing to make sacrifices on their behalf. It just doesn't always have to be the same adult, every single time, every single day. Here, then, is a four-step plan for achieving selfism.

Do one small thing just for yourself. If you're willing and able to spend money on yourself, by all means do so. Take a class or join a gym. Buy yourself a new pair of shoes or have lunch with a friend. Spending some money on yourself is tangible proof—to you, and to your children and husband—that you believe you are worth it.

There's also plenty to do for yourself that's free. Take a brisk walk, go for a bike ride, read a library book. And don't give anyone else the remote. In fact, change channels 25 times every minute, if you want.

Share the sacrifices. Since raising children requires too much work for just one person, fathers have to be willing to take on some of the burden. If your husband doesn't see the truth in this, he may not realize how much you do for your family. Keep a diary for a month, noting every time you make a sacrifice and for whom. Present the evidence to your husband at a quiet moment—not in an accusatory way but simply to offer proof of what you do. Talk with him about which activities seem unnecessary, which to continue, and which he might be able to take on. If he's interested in improving the quality of your marriage and your well-being, he'll give it a try.

Respect yourself. Because self-respect requires a strong inner conviction, it will come gradually once you begin doing more for yourself. Again, acting as if you respect yourself will help you come to feel that you really do. If you do things you like every day, if you spend time focusing on you, you will prove to yourself that you are worthy of respect.

Find a dream. A selfist mother should feel like an essential part of her family. But she should also have a sense of herself as a separate human being, with hopes and desires that belong to her alone. She should have a dream—a realistic vision or goal that she hopes to reach in her lifetime.

A dream is not wanting to become a supermodel or a rock star, because those fantasies are out of the realm of possibility for most of us. A dream is something real, something that will make her feel whole when she achieves it. It can be as clear-cut as going back to school or as undefined as becoming an artist or a horse breeder. To find such a dream, a mother has to go beyond her babies. She has to reach deep down inside and discover who she is and what she wants out of life. This can take a lot of time and effort, but it can also pay the biggest dividends.

part six

Long-Lasting Love

6

Quick Quiz

What's Your Relationship IQ?

Whether you and your partner have been married for years or are in a fairly new relationship, the following quiz—developed by David H. Olson, Ph.D., professor of family social science at the University of Minnesota and president of Life Innovations, both in Minneapolis—will give you some idea of what type of couple you are. Simply mark each statement "yes" or "no," then tally your score as instructed. Keep in mind that the quiz is not designed to predict whether you will have a successful relationship. Rather, it's intended to get you and your partner to talk about important issues.

_____1. I am very pleased with how we support and care for each other. (If you answer no, be sure to read How Do You Make Love Last? on page 246.)

_____2. My partner has some habits that I dislike.

_____3. I can easily share my positive and negative feelings with my partner.

_____4. We have some important disagreements that never seem to get resolved. (Master Your Mate's Moods on page 252 has valuable advice for you.)

_____5. We have decided how to handle our finances.

_____6. At times, I feel pressured to participate in activities that my partner enjoys.

____7. I am very satisfied with the amount of affection that I receive from my partner. (If you answered no to this, you may want to take a peek at The Secrets of Sensual, Satisfying Sex on page 257.)

____8. I have some concerns about how my partner will be as a parent.

____9. We clearly have decided how we will share household responsibilities.

____10. We sometimes disagree on how to practice our religious beliefs.

Interpreting Your Score

Count your yes responses to the odd-numbered questions and your no responses to the even-numbered questions. Then add the two sums together for your total score.

9 or 10. You are a Vitalized Couple. You share many relationship strengths, particularly in communication and understanding each other. Keep up the good work.

6 to 8. You are a Harmonious Couple. You have many strengths, but you could improve some areas of your relationship. You generally have good communication and conflict-resolution skills. You seem to be off to a good start.

4 or 5. You are a Traditional Couple. The two of you are compatible and realistic in how you want to live your life. But you could use some improvement in communication and problem-solving skills.

0 to 3. You are a Conflicted Couple, with many existing or potential relationship difficulties. If the two of you are considering marriage, you may want to seek counseling first.

36

How Do You
Make Love
Last?

Ever wondered, "Do I love him? Really love him?" Of course you have. Every married woman ponders that question sooner or later. In fact, thousands of women pose that question to their family physicians (yes, you read that right), hoping for some professional guidance on a sticky subject. But asking "Do I love my spouse?" is a natural part of any long-term relationship.

According to one national survey, 53 percent of couples rate their love for their partners a "perfect 10." But women make up the smaller part of that happy equation. While 59 percent of men reported that they love their mates with all their hearts, only 47 percent of women said the same. And a full 45 percent of those women wonder, at least sometimes, if they are still in love at all.

Most people say they "fell in love" or describe love as "magic." "But I don't think either is appropriate," says John Gottman, Ph.D., professor of psychology at the University of Washington in Seattle and co-director (with his wife, clinical psychologist Julie Gottman, Ph.D.) of the Seattle Marital and Family Institute. "Based on my research, love is an orderly, systematic process that begins when we decide to turn toward each other and ends when we choose to turn away. Love is, quite simply, a choice we make."

Women Say "I Don't" to Proposing

Equality in marriage seems like a fine proposition. Yet according to a recent survey, proposing marriage is still largely a man's job. Perhaps even more surprising, women are less likely to propose today than they were nearly half a century ago.

A 1997 poll conducted by the Princeton, New Jersey–based Gallup Organization asked 592 randomly selected married adults to identify which spouse had popped the question. Eighty-two percent of the poll participants reported that the husband had done the asking. Only 9 percent said the wife had proposed.

Compare those figures to the results of a similar Gallup poll conducted in 1952. Back then, 76 percent of the poll participants said the husband had proposed, while 12 percent said the wife had. Apparently, women were a little less willing to wait around for men to make the first move.

The 1997 poll revealed another interesting trend: Younger couples are more likely to have gone the traditional route than older couples. Among poll participants under age 30, men had proposed 90 percent of the time; women, 4 percent of the time. Among participants over age 50, the split was 81 percent men, 10 percent women.

Does this mean coyness is making a comeback, at least where proposing is concerned? Probably not, says Leah J. Dickstein, M.D., professor and associate chairman for academic affairs in the department of psychiatry and behavioral sciences at the University of Louisville School of Medicine in Kentucky. She speculates that greater financial security and a high divorce rate have left women shy not of proposing but of marriage itself. "In general, many women value their independence and are not rushing into marriage," she observes.

Marriage under a Microscope

In his Seattle "laboratory"—actually, an apartment—Dr. Gottman has filmed literally hundreds of couples going about the business of their daily lives: eating, reading, relaxing, communicating, quarreling, the works. He has recorded even the most minute changes in their facial expressions, body language, blood pressures, and sweat rates during both emotional and what he calls neutral interactions. And based on what he has seen and heard, he has developed a methodology for making love stay.

Dr. Gottman's system has nothing to do with magic. Or passion. Or time-outs. Or even that incredibly awkward exercise in which you have to practice "active listening" by patiently repeating what your partner has just barked at you. More basic and less labored than that, it has to do mostly with friendship.

"Once you enhance the friendship within your marriage, you don't have a chip on your shoulder when your partner is in a crabby mood," says Dr. Gottman, who is also author of *Why Marriages Succeed or Fail*. "Let's just say you have enough emotional money in the bank, so the conflicts that arise between you aren't disabling."

Everyone knows cash can't buy happiness. What few people realize, however, is that emotional money just may buy you a happy marriage.

A State of Temporary Insanity

Sociologists have long studied the process of falling in . . . er, make that finding love. And they've found that perceived similarity is a predictor of love. "If you think someone may be like you, you're attracted to that person, you start thinking a lot about that person, and that's what people call being in love," says Dr. Gottman. "But that's also part of what makes love so dangerous—the fact that it's based on perceptions and that our perceptions aren't always accurate." Especially given how most couples cozy up to one another when courting.

"I like to call being in love a form of temporary insanity," says Marjorie Hansen Shaevitz, director of the Institute for Family and Work Relationships in La Jolla, California. "What you tend to do is basically ignore everything that you don't want to see in the other person. And you show that person everything that you want him to see about you."

This occurs even among folks who are supposed to know better—including Hansen Shaevitz and her husband, Mort, also a clinical psychologist. "Mort is brilliant in the office," says Hansen Shaevitz. "At home, he's just a regular man. He has all of these resources and skills and qualities—they're the reasons I fell in love with him, really. But especially in the early years of our marriage, he didn't use those skills with me. At first, when we were dating, he was just nuts about me. He would have done anything for me. But shortly after we were married, he would come home and just read the newspaper. He shut down."

Hansen Shaevitz figured the best way to reshape her new husband's behavior was to work on the issue together, as professionals. So she suggested that they write a book on two-career couples, a novel phenomenon back in the mid-1970s. The result was *Making It Together As a Two-Career Couple*, but still the same old Mort.

"So then I wrote a book called *The Superwoman Syndrome* because I was still trying to do it all," says Hansen Shaevitz. And Mort? "He wrote *Sexual Static: How Men Are Confusing the Women They Love.*"

Getting to Know You

Not getting to know the real person behind a romantic partner can spell trouble for any marriage—unless, that is, the lovers happen to also be friends. "We've been studying 130 newlywed couples," says Dr. Gottman. "We found that in 75 percent of the couples, the wife's marital satisfaction plummeted when the first baby arrived. In 25 percent, it didn't—in fact, sometimes it went up. So we tried to pinpoint the difference between the happy and unhappy couples. And we found that the happy couples knew about each other's psychological worlds, about their partners' worries, hopes, and dreams. They were friends. They were attentive to what was happening in each other's lives, just as friends would be. And that made all the difference in their marriages."

Lexi and Jim had been married for nearly three years when their daughter, Angela, arrived. "When I first started staying home with Angela, Jim would ask how my day went when he walked in the door, and I'd say 'I got three loads of laundry done!'" Lexi laughs. "Yet he'd be excited for me—really. And I love that. Because even when nothing big happens, you still want to share the day's tiny triumphs and traumas with your partner. You want him to know what your everyday life is like. You want him to live it with you."

Dr. Gottman's insights into newlyweds' postbaby blues led him and his wife to develop a board game, which they require all couples who attend their institute to play. The only way to advance within the game? By correctly answering what some might consider nitpicky questions about your partner's life and loves.

- ❖ At what age does he aim to retire?
- ❖ Did he always plan to be in his current line of work?
- ❖ What's the biggest item on his professional plate in the next month?
- ❖ What's his favorite sports team? Are they doing well?
- ❖ How did his family demonstrate love?

"Friends know stuff like this about each other," says Dr. Gottman. "They have cognitive room for their friends' feelings, so they can be very giving. They ask questions of each other and keep in touch. That is why couples who base their love on friendship have a much better shot than those who base their love on a perception."

Your Emotional Bank Account

When couples in marital therapy argue, they're often asked to practice what some psychologists and self-help texts call active listening. Dr. Gottman advises against it. "Tell me," he asks, "who can act compassionate when they're feeling attacked?"

Instead, what Dr. Gottman advocates is a form of active listening during neutral moments, like when you're eating together, driving together, even checking in on each other by phone. As illogical as it may seem, you build your emotional bank account during such nonemotional moments.

Linda and Steve, married for 11 years, have built a hefty emotional nest egg— even though Linda describes her husband as "quiet, someone who isn't always comfortable emoting." But Steve figured out a way to make Linda feel loved and listened to: He leaves funny messages for her on their answering machine.

"I'll get, 'Hello, this is the Publishers Clearing House Prize Patrol calling. Can you give us directions to your house?' when we've just spent the evening filling out one of those things," says Linda. "I love that he does it. It's his way of letting me know that he's thinking about me during the day. And the messages just crack me up." As a result, Linda feels rich in love, but so does Steve because he gets his wife's attention.

"A couple's emotional bank account can be very tough to gauge unless you have a laboratory like mine, where couples share the same mundane routine— like eating together or reading the newspaper together—that they would at home," says Dr. Gottman. "As a result, we have hundreds of hours of videotape of people making bids for attention. That's what we do all day—make bids for attention. We ask questions, comment on current events, point out curiosities in the landscape. Some partners respond to our bids with interest, meaning that they turn toward us. Others only grudgingly reply or don't even answer." This turning away may cause a person to wonder, "Do I really love my spouse?"

After analyzing the videotape of a couple interacting in his lab, Dr. Gottman compares the number of times they turn toward each other with the number of times they turn away from each other. "We actually compute a ratio by dividing the number of times a couple turn toward each other by the total number of bids for attention," Dr. Gottman explains. "What we've found is that in marriages that are going well, there's a very high ratio of turning toward each other. These people tend to want to hear what their partners find interesting."

And not just on pulse points, such as abortion, politics, and religion, but during nonemotional moments, too. "By and large, these bids for attention occur during mindless moments, when you're on autopilot," says Dr. Gottman. "Yet they're more critical than you might think. Over the course of a marriage, you endure literally thousands of them. And what they're communicating is real interest in your partner." Or, of course, a lack thereof.

Eileen and Bob have been married for 12 years and have been together as friends for 15. "I'm pretty affectionate," says Eileen. "So if Bob is reading the newspaper and I want to talk to him, I usually wrap my arms around him from the back and caress him. Sometimes I'll look over his shoulder and ask him if he's reading something really interesting. I'll go with him where he's going, and in most cases, he responds by welcoming me there. Every now and then, he'll get a little annoyed. But generally, he'll look up and make eye contact. Then we'll move from what's in the paper to what went on in his day and what happened during mine."

Five-Minute Moments

At the Seattle Marital and Family Institute, the Gottmans encourage couples to take mindless moments and make them mindful. "You would never ignore a close friend's bid for interest or attention," says Dr. Gottman. "Funny how all bets are off when you start sleeping with someone."

Maureen and Michael have been together for 13 years, married for 6. Their first child, Julia, arrived a few months ago. "There's one thing Michael does that I love," says Maureen. "He always kisses me first—even before he kisses the baby—when he walks in the door at the end of the day. His parents always put their kids before their relationship, and they ended up sacrificing their marriage as a result. So it's a conscious choice of Michael's to put his relationship with me first. Our marriage is fulfilling now and will continue to be, long after Julia is grown and gone."

It's these little things—the five-minute moments, says Dr. Gottman—that count. As part of their campaign to get couples accustomed to thinking as teammates, the Gottmans suggest that partners take five minutes every morning to find out one important thing that will happen during the course of the other's day. "For instance, when I hear that my wife is joining our friend Jean for lunch, I find myself wondering right around lunchtime what the two of them are doing, where they're eating, how it's going," says Dr. Gottman. "And I usually remember to ask my wife about it later."

Margaret, a nurse, can relate. "As goofy as it sounds, I really love telling Rudi about my day," she says of her husband of four years. "I work 12-hour shifts, so he's usually home by the time I roll through the door. And the first thing he asks me is 'How was your day?' A lot of times, he even remembers the names of my patients, and he'll ask, 'How is so-and-so doing? How did his surgery go? How's his breathing?' He pays attention to my life. That's a big part of what drew me to him, actually. He listens to me—and he likes it."

"All the parts of love—the passion, the romance—they flow from friendship," says Dr. Gottman. "So what we've done is take the magic that exists in good friendships and break it down to make it accessible to everyone." Even husbands and wives.

"I'm a passionate woman, and it feels fantastic to be so passionate after all these years," says Eileen. "I've always felt that the passion comes from deep friendship. And the passion between us is stronger than ever. I know it's because we trust and respect each other more than we did the day we got married. Our friendship has deepened."

37

Master Your Mate's Moods

W*e're packing up the car for a picnic. I've made cucumber sandwiches and blueberry pie. Dark silver clouds border one edge of the sky, but the weatherman says they'll clear. It should be a perfect day, except Peter is in one of his moods. He's muttering gloomy pronouncements about the day, like "It'll probably rain—we'll have to leave as soon as we get to the park." Then I ask him to put on Katie's shoes. She does that two-year-old thing, kicking like a wild thing and whining. Peter throws her sandals down on the ground and says, "She doesn't want anything to do with me! She only wants you these days." Then huffs off down the driveway. An hour before, he had been in a perfectly good mood. What's his problem?*

—Sally, a working mother of two in Seattle

The answer to that question would be simple ("He's a jerk!") if Peter were always this moody and negative. But he's not. He happens to be a warm listener and a perceptive and supportive friend to Sally. When they aren't being visited by one of Peter's black moods, Sally is happy—with Peter and with their marriage.

But "the mood" always returns when Sally least expects it, like an unwelcome houseguest. Its recurring presence has worn her down. Sound familiar? If you're like many couples, you're dying for a solution to this common complaint.

Partners in Pain

A wife may be more sensitive to her husband's pain than he is to hers, suggests a recent study of osteoarthritis patients conducted at Duke University in Durham, North Carolina. Watching tapes of the patients performing a variety of tasks, women were more accurate in detecting the level of pain reported by their husbands than vice versa. "It may be that women are more tuned in to picking up social cues in people than men are," says Francis Keefe, Ph.D., professor at Ohio University in Athens and one of the researchers in the study.

If your spouse suffers from chronic pain, you can help simply by letting him vent about his discomfort. Ask him questions rather than offering solutions. And work together to map out his pain cycles, so you can predict when a flare-up is about to hit and take steps to prevent or alleviate it.

What Is Moody, Anyway?

We all have myriad moods, highs and lows. But if your mate doesn't seem able to manage or control his moods—meaning he can't yank himself out of them, redirect his thoughts, or tell someone how he's feeling in a way that brings relief—and they often shift out of control, he probably falls into a category called mood lability (meaning changeability). These are people who tend to be very overreactive, who respond in a rush of feeling to almost anything going on around them, says John Ratey, M.D., assistant professor of psychiatry at Harvard Medical School. On the bright side, along with that big bundle of overly sensitive nerves comes a big plus: Like Peter, most moody men can tune in to and empathize with your emotions better than other men do.

But when in a funk, a moody man's personality takes a decidedly male turn for the worse. Women with mood lability usually become sad, withdrawn, down. Men are more likely to lash out. Following are the most common manifestations of men's bad moods.

The tantrum thrower. Sally says that the last time she and Peter had "an incident," he was putting a tricycle together for their son's third birthday. Peter had spent hours working on it, only to realize that the store had given him the wrong screws. "I told him, 'Take it back to the store. It's no big deal,'" Sally recalls. "But it sent him into this scowling, dark tizzy for an hour. Finally, he found some screws that fit and put the tricycle together. We took Sam outside to see it, but he didn't feel like riding it. So Peter stalked off, saying 'That was my whole stinking day!' I hate the example his tantrums set for our kids."

The angry critic. A close cousin to the guy who makes a scene is the one who becomes irritable, argumentative, and critical of you. Take Max, a financial analyst living in Boston. Max is pretty forthcoming about his moods and admits, "Little things throw me off kilter. Like one night, my girlfriend, Gay, whom I live with, wanted us to go over the phone bill together. But being asked about it when I was so tired from work just set me off, and I snapped at her in the most condescending way: 'Listen, Gay, can't you figure it out yourself?' The thing is, it's not really what I say, it's that I get this tone that sounds as if I'm really putting her down."

The refrigerator. Mike says that "being set off" doesn't make him strike out. Instead, he aggressively withdraws. "Say I'm immersed in working on my boat and my wife, Amy, interrupts me, wanting an answer about something I'm not ready to give an answer on. I'll retreat and shut down—just not look at her, or even walk away. I usually need a break to chill out, get off by myself, before I'm able to have a real conversation."

The moper. George also withdraws, but without any attendant relief. "If someone at the agency where I work says something I perceive to be derogatory, I'll go over and over it in my mind until I feel this cosmic despair that is way out of proportion," he says. "I feel as if I'm trapped in a cave and can't even reach out to my wife." Jackie, a marketing executive, says she can see one of George's moods coming a mile away: "The first sign is that he'll say, 'I'm dizzy' or 'I'm very tired.' Then he turns very negative and uses a lot of profanity. Sometimes he'll try to pin his mood on me. He'll imply that it's my fault—that I don't love him enough, and that's why he's in a funk."

So What Causes These Moods?

The reasons for moodiness are as complicated as your mercurial mate. According to Robert Thayer, Ph.D., author of *The Origin of Everyday Moods: Managing Energy, Tension, and Stress*, all of our moods—both bad and good—are tightly tied to our physical states. How we're feeling physically interacts with our thoughts to produce our moods. In other words, just as we are likely to be in a good mood when we feel high energy and little tension, we will probably be in a funk when we have low physical energy and moderately high tension. Some people, of course, are more anxiety-prone or less energetic than others. It's essential, then, to tune in to those states and begin to learn how to keep a balance.

Evidence also suggests that some people are simply hardwired to occasionally go haywire. PET (positron-emission tomography) scans, which provide detailed pictures of the brain as it functions, show that some adults with mood lability may have a defect in the cortex, the part of the brain responsible for executive decision-making. When people with this condition, called hypofrontality, are deciding how to behave in emotionally trying situations, the frontal lobes of the brain's cortex don't register a normal amount of activity. "The major job of the brain's cortex is to put the brakes on impulsive behavior, temper tantrums, and so on," explains Dr. Ratey, who is also co-author of the book *Shadow Syndromes*. "Most of us talk ourselves out of a mood because, even as we're acting impulsively, we're thinking about the ramifications of our behavior. But those with hypofrontality can't do that. They behave in destructive ways because they can't stop to consider what the consequences of their actions will be."

PET scans have also shown that people with severe moodiness often suffer from a lack of the brain chemical serotonin. "The link between low serotonin and aggressive moods is profound," Dr. Ratey says. And if a person's moodiness interferes with love and work enough, it may be necessary to increase levels of serotonin, often with antidepressants such as fluoxetine (Prozac).

Nix the Negativity

So what are you supposed to do about all this? If you're at your wits' end and contemplating drastic measures—electroshock therapy, maybe?—take heart. There are simpler ways to live harmoniously with these guys, even change them.

Next time you sense that your partner is shifting into his less-than-lovely self, try these eight strategies gleaned from experts and moody men themselves. We hope they'll put you both in a better mood.

Find his mood triggers. Try to identify what's unique about the times that he's down or angry—and what's going on when he's not, advises Michele Weiner-Davis, author of *Divorce Busting*. Some women report that their men are easily set off when they haven't eaten recently. Other women say that when their mates are keeping any type of secret (like making a golf date on your anniversary), they "act out" their guilt by moping around. After recognizing a pattern, you can both work to break it.

Take a moment to chill. Time alone is a rarity. So let him have his time tinkering in the garage or reading the sports section—and use it to do your own thing.

Try to let little things go. "I think the worst advice any woman can get is to discuss *every* feeling," Weiner-Davis says. "If you call him on every transgression, you're going to find that doing so often escalates the scene into something even uglier. If you let it go, on the other hand, you may well go on to have a perfectly lovely day."

Get a grip on your anxiety. Of course, letting go of little stuff would be a lot easier if you didn't feel so anxious when your mate grows irritable: What if your kids are scarred by his shifting highs and lows? Why should you have to deal with his mood problems one more time? "Remind yourself that you're staying nonreactive for your own sake, not his," Weiner-Davis advises. "You want to improve the quality of your life, you want to have a good day, and you don't want him to ruin it." And if you do end up telling him to take a hike? Don't sweat it, Weiner-Davis says. Remember, tomorrow is another day.

Reverse directions. Weiner-Davis tells the story of a woman named Rebecca, whose husband, Joe, would come home so upset he'd bang his fists on the dinner table as he told her about work. Rebecca's natural response was to say, "It will be all right, honey, really." Then Joe would get even madder at her for not understanding his angst. So she'd get angry and yell, "I'm trying to help! How can you get mad at me?" But when Rebecca once tried saying, "Oh, that is awful," Joe calmed right down. In fact, he even said, "I'm probably exaggerating."

Many men agree that the worst thing you can do is try to cajole, brush away, or make light of their bad moods. "When she blithely says, 'Oh, come on! Let's go for a walk! You'll feel better!' I feel she's implying I don't have a valid reason to feel bad," George says.

Try gentle questioning. When he starts withdrawing into a long, blue funk, try reaching out with a few loving questions, says Laura Epstein Rosen, Ph.D., co-author of *When Someone You Love Is Depressed*. Leading questions are best: "Are you feeling worried about work?" or "Are you feeling tense about your mother visiting tomorrow?" You may not hit the nail on the head. But as Dr. Rosen notes, this might open up a dialogue—a critical part of lifting him out of his foul mood. If you can't, and if his moods remain low and constant, they might signal depression. In that case, your mate should see a doctor.

Inject a little humor. "Women often overlook humor as a tool for dealing with moodiness," says Weiner-Davis. "Yet it can be very effective." So crack a joke—it might crack his black mood, too.

Reevaluate your relationship. Suppose none of the above makes even the slightest dent in your days and nights with this man. You do, at a certain point, have to ask yourself if it's all worth it. If he still denies that he has a problem— even when you call him only on the big, unforgivable stuff—and it goes on unchecked for months, you and your mate may need to go your separate ways. And if the situation turns emotionally or physically abusive, absolutely leave at once and get yourself and your children to safety.

38

The Secrets of Sensual, Satisfying Sex

E llen was roaming the aisles of her local Sears store, trying frantically to keep track of her three youngsters while her mother did some shopping. At least her mom knew exactly what she wanted. She made a beeline for the sporting goods aisle, where she began strapping on ankle weights.

"What's this all about?" Ellen wanted to know.

"Oh, it's just a new way to stay in shape," her mother replied. Then, after looking around to see whether any grandchildren were in earshot, she confided a secret motivation. "You know, dear, your father is a very virile man."

"Oh, great," Ellen thought. It was bad enough that her own love life with her husband, Doug, had tapered off. Of course, she felt guilty about that, but she had always blamed it on their hectic lifestyle. Her mother's casual remark made her stop denying the problem. "My mom is nearly 70," Ellen said later, "and her sex life is probably better than mine!"

Romance on the Rocks

If you're having a sexual midlife crisis, you may feel alone, at wit's end, and unable to talk about it. What's more, the sexual anecdotes your girlfriend shares with you on Monday morning may make you feel as though other women couldn't commiserate. Oh, but they could: Polls have shown that while 85 per-

Sex-Induced Amnesia

This might be the most novel excuse for forgetting a partner's name after a passionate tryst: intercourse-induced amnesia.

In a letter to a British medical journal, Dr. Russell Lane, a neurologist at Charing Cross Hospital in London, recounted the case of a 64-year-old man whose wife reported that he had experienced sex-linked memory loss on five separate occasions over an 18-month period. In his confused state, the man repeatedly asked, "What are we doing?" and "What time of day is it?" Afterward, he couldn't remember making love and had only a fuzzy recollection of foreplay.

This is not exactly news that thrills a spouse, so the couple sought Dr. Lane's advice. He learned that the man had a 20-year history of migraine headaches—including some triggered by sex. And an examination of the man's brain waves revealed some abnormal activity.

Dr. Lane concluded that his patient had probably experienced a phenomenon known as transient global amnesia. The exact cause of the condition, which typically affects folks ages 50 and older, hasn't been nailed down. But migraines seem to be a common thread, according to Dr. John Hodges, a neurologist at Cambridge University who's an expert on memory disorders. A wide variety of physical and emotional stressors are known to prompt these brief bouts of amnesia, Dr. Hodges says. Coitus accounts for about 5 percent of all cases.

But a cold shower isn't the answer. "Sometimes the syndrome is called amnesia-by-the-seaside," Dr. Hodges notes, "because older people who suddenly go for a swim in very cold water can have an attack."

HEALTH FLASH

cent of women are satisfied with their marriages, only 57 percent are satisfied with their sex lives.

A major culprit is—no surprise—the pace of life in the 1990s. "Day-to-day stress prevents women from being romantic and feeling responsive to a man's advances," observes John Gray, Ph.D., author of *Men Are from Mars, Women Are from Venus.* "It just gets worse every day. Life is only speeding up." And under these conditions, he says, "Love alone will not create romance."

To be sure, how often you have sex may decrease as you get older. One large survey of Americans' sexual practices found that frequency of sex was highest among men and women in their late twenties, 47 percent of whom said they enjoyed sex two or more times a week. By comparison, more than 40 percent of women in their fifties reported that they hadn't had sex in the previous year.

There are some age-old reasons for this. For one, you're not being driven by a surge of teenage hormones anymore. For another, the novelty wears off. Because of what psychologists call habituation, a marriage can become less sexy even as it grows more comfortable each year. Patricia Love, Ed.D., author of *Hot Monogamy*, has a colorful way of putting it: "If you live by the railroad tracks and a train goes by, you don't even wake up."

But the complexities of modern life serve to make matters worse. Couples like Ellen and Doug have to cope with two jobs, three kids, four seasons' worth of sports leagues, and a multitude of responsibilities in the new, downsized workplace. Millions of Americans are feeling the effects of "time famine." Put simply, they are starved for an open half-hour.

Too Busy, Too Tired

According to Sheryl Kingsberg, Ph.D., assistant professor of obstetrics/gynecology and psychology at Case Western Reserve University in Cleveland, a threat to healthy marital relations can occur not just at midlife but any time external distractions start to mount up. She wouldn't be surprised if some couples with young children are not having as much fun as their vivacious retired parents. "My sense is, as couples get older, they have more time. So their sexual relations can actually improve."

At Canyon Ranch, a spa in Tucson, Arizona, stressed-out couples can enroll in a four-day workshop called Sex: Body and Soul. Their very first task is to identify what they think has gotten in the way of their sex lives. "The number one answer is 'too busy and too tired,'" reports Lana Holstein, M.D., who leads the workshop with her husband, David Taylor, M.D., and is director of women's health at Canyon Ranch. "That's what comes up over and over again. I see more celibate couples now than I've ever seen." No, these people haven't taken vows to keep their hands off each other. But they may as well, considering that their erotic escapades have dwindled to perhaps three or four per year.

Too tired, indeed. A busy, stressful life can leave you just plain physically exhausted. Almost 100 million Americans don't get enough sleep at night, and one-quarter of the nation's workforce labors through the evening, says Michael A. Perelman, Ph.D., a clinical psychologist and co-director of the Human Sexuality Program at New York Hospital in Manhattan. In fact, Dr. Perelman, who specializes in sex and marital therapy, believes that fatigue is probably the number one cause of sexual distress in the United States.

Sex Is Not Just Sex

For some couples, infrequent sex is not a problem. Their reaction may be to shrug and ask, "So what?" And as long as both partners agree, that's their business.

But for most couples, the fact that you haven't been intimate for six months is not quite the same as, say, the fact that you haven't gone hiking together since last summer. A relationship doesn't grow frayed and testy from a lack of trail-blazing. But it may well wither from a lack of sex. "Sex is not just sex," says Bernie Zilbergeld, Ph.D., a sex therapist in Oakland, California, and author of *The New Male Sexuality*. "It's a major glue that keeps two people together."

Indeed, studies of happy marriages find a lot of happy moments behind closed doors. "A good sex life, however the couple defines that, is at the heart of a good marriage," says clinical psychologist Judith Wallerstein in her book *The Good Marriage: How and Why Love Lasts*. The book is based on her study of 50 happily married couples and draws upon their experiences to distill nine fundamental characteristics of a good marriage. Sexual love is among them. "This is the domain where intimacy is renewed, and the excitement that first drew the couple together is kept alive," Wallerstein writes. "There is no better antidote to the pressures of living than a loving sex life."

This sounds wonderful—but for most of us, it's easier said than done. Most sex therapists recognize that getting "unstuck" from a sexual slump is difficult and that the process by which a couple reconnects with each other may require the hashing out of many issues. The first step is for both partners to acknowledge the problem—an acknowledgment that may begin with saying something simple and straight from the heart.

Ways to Fan the Flame

The good news is that when couples do take the time and make the effort to rediscover their sexual attraction, they are in for a very pleasant surprise. "The best sex happens between couples who have been together a long time," Dr. Holstein notes. "It's better to have a foundation of commitment and emotional intimacy with an atmosphere of truth-telling than to have high hormone levels."

When you're both ready to start rekindling those old flames, here are some incendiary devices.

Make it important. "Most marriages die of neglect," Dr. Love says. The union slowly erodes, and neither partner knows how to get it back where it was. Sex is one way to reignite a relationship, but sex won't happen without first honoring its importance. One of Dr. Love's clients drew up a document—it actually looked like a legal agreement—in which she promised her husband that she'd be a better lover. "She knew she had a good marriage, and she wanted to protect it," Dr. Love recalls. "She was smart. Her only problem was, she had no idea how!" But at least she had taken that key first step. Competent sex therapy can help with the details. Unfortunately, Dr. Love says, she sees many couples who have an unwritten contract that's a recipe for disaster. It says, in effect, "I expect you to be monogamous, but don't expect me to meet your sexual needs."

Make time and space. "There are people who have the same miserable schedule you do, and they are having sex," Dr. Zilbergeld observes. "They put sex higher on the list." There's a time and place for everything—but, of course, you have to find the time and place. "People bridle at this," he says. "They'll say, 'I hate to schedule time for sex.' Well, the world is on a schedule. I'm all for spontaneity—but the problem is, in a life that's completely scheduled, whatever is not scheduled will fall through the cracks." So when he counsels couples, an hour of therapy will often end with two people getting out their separate but equally fat appointment books and making a date.

Get out of town. In his book *Mars and Venus in the Bedroom: A Guide to Lasting Romance and Passion*, Dr. Gray says the primary reason why some couples lose interest in sex is that the man feels rejected and the woman doesn't feel romanced and understood. It can become a vicious circle, and stress only exacerbates it. "Ironically, as we have more technological advances and conveniences, women are busier," he explains. "They use the time to take on more obligations and responsibilities. The more stressed they get, the more they're unable to relax. So the question is: How do you get a woman to stop and relax? The only thing that will do it is romance."

And that means getting out of town. "For a woman to feel special, you need to have special occasions," he says. "You have to deliberately create time away from stressful situations, from kids, from work. A woman has to be taken out of the stressful environment. This will allow her to feel like herself again. It takes her back to her center—back to her loving, compassionate self. In a busy, busy world, romance is the only thing that can take her back."

As for the rejected husband, "when he gets her in that place, he, too, will feel romantic again," Dr. Gray says. "Her responsiveness will stimulate him, and he will become aroused."

Not every couple can run off to Bali for a week, as Dr. Gray and his wife, Bonnie, once did. But more couples could do something else the Grays do: Go away overnight once a month. "It has to be just her and me, no kids and no work, for at least 24 hours," he says. "And nobody can intrude."

Treat sex like exercise. With sex, as with exercise, you don't necessarily want to do it when you first start out. But you know that you should. And you know that by the end, you'll feel better. So you have to be willing to start a sexual connection from zero, or even minus one, on the scale of desire. Once you have made love, you are usually glad you did—just like exercise.

Let's Get Physical

Exercise is sexy for lots of reasons (behold spandex shorts). But here's the best yet: An aerobic workout—even a brief one—can help put you in the mood for love and even give your orgasms more punch, says Linda DeVillers, Ph.D., a sex therapist in El Segundo, California, and author of *Love Skills*.

"Aerobic exercise increases activity in the left frontal lobe of the brain, triggering positive feelings that can boost interest in sex," Dr. DeVillers says, citing research from Arizona State University in Tempe. Exercise also triggers production of feel-good chemicals called endorphins, which can increase not only your arousal but possibly the intensity of your orgasms as well. "The effect lasts for 60 to 90 minutes after 10 minutes or more of activity," Dr. DeVillers notes. Consider mentioning this tidbit to your sweetie.

This may seem like work, but it isn't. And let's face it: You need something to replace the magical attraction from your courtship days. "People assume that something is wrong if you have to work at romance," Dr. Kingsberg says. "In fact, it's required."

Actually get some exercise. As you get older, the role of exercise becomes critical in maintaining sexual desire, physical energy, and self-esteem. In fact, exercise can work like an aphrodisiac to improve your sex life. Recently, scientists at the University of California, San Diego, conducted a nine-month study of 78 sedentary people. By the end of the study, the people who were put through some serious aerobic training for one hour every other day were making love 30 percent more often than people who were less active.

Stop being Martha Stewart. For all of the talk here about having to work at romance, please don't go overboard. "For many people, there are only two kinds of sex—perfect sex and no sex at all," says Judith Seifer, Ph.D., co-creator and host of the *Better Sex* video series. "When I say any sex is better than no sex at all, people don't believe me." She gets rankled when she hears people refer to her as "the Martha Stewart of sex." Her intent is to help couples improve their sex lives, not to elevate it to some state of fussed-over perfection.

In her role as sex therapist, Dr. Seifer finds that couples tend to focus on what's wrong with their sex lives instead of trying to build upon what's right. She says she ends up telling them, "I don't want quality over quantity. That's what has gotten you to the point where you're sitting in my office today." She suggests that they get rid of what she calls perfect-sex syndrome.

part seven

Beauty Secrets for Busy Women

7

Quick Quiz

Do You Know Your Beauty Basics?

If you're like many women, you've probably followed pretty much the same beauty routine for years. You know what works, and you know what you're comfortable with.

Still, your routine may be in need of some updating—especially if you've based it on certain beauty myths. Can you spot them in the following list? Simply mark each statement "true" or "false," then check your responses against those at the end of the quiz.

_____1. Facial exercises erase wrinkles and keep skin smooth.

_____2. Sleeping on your side or stomach causes wrinkles.

_____3. Placing tea bags over your eyes helps reduce puffiness.

_____4. Tanning beds are a safe alternative to direct sunlight.

_____5. You should throw away any cosmetics that you haven't used in three years.

_____6. You can make your hair grow faster by massaging your scalp.

_____7. Certain shampoos can actually make your hair appear thicker.

_____8. Losing up to 100 hairs a day is perfectly normal for women.

Answers

1. False. Yes, many books and magazines tout facial exercises. But the fact is that repeatedly contorting your face in the same way creates wrinkles rather than erasing them. (If you want to keep your skin looking young and healthy, see Look Your Best at Any Age on page 266.)

2. True. The creases in the pillowcase press against your face, causing wrinkles. Yes, they're only temporary—but as you get older, they can last well into the day. You're better off sleeping on your back. If you find that position uncomfortable, try using a satin pillowcase instead.

3. True. Chamomile and green teas have properties that effectively eliminate puffiness around the eyes. Just steep the tea bags and allow them to cool. Then place them over your eyes for up to five minutes. (For other home remedies, take a peek at Fast Fixes for Tired Eyes on page 273.)

4. False. In fact, some experts argue that lying in a tanning bed is even more dangerous than lying out in the sun. One reason: Tanning lamps generate more than five times the ultraviolet radiation that you'd be exposed to if you were sitting on a beach at the equator. If you really want a "healthy glow," try one of the new self tanning lotions

5. True . . . with an asterisk. Actually, you should throw away all cosmetics after one year, regardless of whether you're using them. When they're that old, they can harbor harmful germs and microbes. (For specifics on what to toss when, turn to Apply Makeup Like a Pro on page 281.)

6. False. Your hair grows at a rate of about one-half inch a month, regardless of whether you massage your scalp. Nevertheless, doing so can make you feel good all over. (To massage your scalp while you shampoo, follow the technique that's described in Fuss-Free Care for Fabulous Hair on page 277.)

7. True. Certain shampoos can coat the hair shaft to make it appear fuller and thicker. Look for a product that is protein-based. The label will likely say something like "body-building" or "volumizing."

8. True. The average woman loses between 50 and 100 hairs a day—which isn't bad, considering you have more than 100,000 hairs on your head. If you think that you're experiencing more severe hair loss, see your doctor.

39

Look Your Best at Any Age

Aging is one of life's harshest realities. Like it or not, we live in a culture where the thought of growing (and looking) old inspires fear, loathing, and insecurity. Where the terms "thirtysomething" and "forty-ish" are accepted without irony. Where $4 billion was spent on anti-aging products in one year alone.

We also live in a country where, by the year 2000, one in three people will be over age 50. That's a lot of women trying to stop the clock.

We may slather ourselves with sunblock, cover up the gray, and opt for a peel here or a brow lift there in an effort to preserve the smooth perkiness of youth. But science may also have an explanation for our behavior.

"Early in our history, when men were looking for mates to eternalize their genes, they looked for youth—smooth skin, shiny hair, and full lips," says Deborah Blum, author of *Sex on the Brain: The Biological Differences between Men and Women.* "Men are predisposed to find those qualities attractive, and we're stuck with it."

Los Angeles social psychologist Debbie Then, Ph.D., offers a contemporary angle. "Vanity is a social reality that stems from a double standard," she says. "Looks and age are intertwined with everything you are as a woman. But it is always to your benefit to look as good as you can."

Of course, as Dr. Then points out, women need to realize that there's more to life than looks. "Don't ruminate about it," she says. "Just do something about it."

An Estrogen Benefit That's Skin Deep

Postmenopausal women may use hormone replacement therapy (HRT) for a variety of reasons—to douse hot flashes, combat vaginal dryness, or ward off heart disease and osteoporosis, for example. They may not know it yet, but their skin may be benefiting as well.

Researchers at the University of California, San Francisco, and the University of California, Los Angeles, examined the skin of more than 3,800 postmenopausal women, most of whom were white. The odds of having wrinkled skin were 32 percent lower in women who began taking estrogen at menopause. For these women, the odds for having dry skin were 24 percent lower.

"Estrogen preserves skin collagen content and thickness, so it makes sense that replacing the hormone in postmenopausal women would help," says Stuart H. Kaplan, M.D., a dermatologist whose private practice in Beverly Hills, California, specializes in cosmetic dermatology. Collagen is a fibrous protein that gives skin its elasticity. It helps to reduce the appearance of fine lines and wrinkles and to relieve excessive dryness. For older women, in particular, excessively dry skin can cause persistent itching and scratching, which increases their risk for infections and pressure sores.

HRT is appropriate only for postmenopausal women with reduced estrogen levels, not for younger women, Dr. Kaplan warns. Using HRT will not improve the skin of a woman with healthy estrogen levels. In fact, it may upset her hormonal balance. For more information about HRT, talk to your gynecologist, internist, or endocrinologist.

Or don't. "I love the wrinkles in Georgia O'Keeffe's face," says New York City makeup artist Francois Nars. "But I love Cher, too. It's whatever makes you happy." And luckily, it seems that happiness comes easier with age.

In the following pages, we'll look closely and candidly at what happens to a woman's skin and self-image at 20, 30, 40, and 50. We hope to dispel some anxiety—and to spell out what a woman can do to look her best at every age.

Twenties: Time Is on Your Side

In her twenties, a woman has a few minor beauty concerns—the occasional zit, puffy eyes after a late night, a bad haircut. She also has one major concern: figuring out who she is and, consequently, what she wants to look like.

Smooth Out Wrinkles

It's not just stress that puts those frown lines between your brows. Grimacing in your sleep or scrunching your face against your pillow can make them look worse, says Dee Anna Glaser, M.D., assistant professor of dermatology at St. Louis University School of Medicine.

To awaken with a smoother forehead, apply surgical tape over the wrinkles before you go to bed. You can also use this trick during the day, when you're home alone. Although it won't erase the wrinkles you already have, the tape will help prevent further furrows by serving as a noticeable, physical reminder when you unconsciously scrunch your brows. (If you notice any redness or irritation from the tape, discontinue use.)

"The early twenties are the fun years," says New York City makeup artist Brigitte Reiss-Andersen. But from age 25 on, things get tougher. "This is when you choose your peers and your profession," notes Reiss-Andersen. "Whether you're a student, a junior executive, or a mother, you're designing your look so that peers can recognize you."

In fact, the predominant worry of a woman in her twenties is that "you have to look sexy to attract the opposite sex, but you're still forging a professional life," observes Dr. Then. "Blending those two looks is really important."

And often really difficult. "Younger people are always more unhappy with their looks because they're particularly susceptible to the illusion that we can be perfect," says Joni Johnston, Psy.D., a clinical psychologist with the Growth Company in San Diego. "When I was in my twenties, I was horrified by the thought of lines. It's funny how little I care about them now that I have them."

The flip side to that pressure to be flawless is the freedom to experiment. "I have this theory that when you're young, makeup is tribal," says makeup artist Mary Greenwell. "You show what you stand for with it—whether you're Gothic with dark eyes and nails, a disco girl with perfect bright red nails, or sporty and very natural." In other words, makeup plays a part, however small, in shaping—and showcasing—a woman's identity.

As for facing the future, the experts have one word of wisdom: prevention. Guzzling water, getting enough sleep, and not drinking alcohol or smoking can keep skin smoother longer. "Wear sunscreen and take your makeup off before you go to sleep," advises Reiss-Andersen. Ah, the simplicity.

Your skin: As far as a woman's complexion goes, this is as good as it gets. Skin cells are rising from deep within the top layer of skin (the epidermis) to the surface (the stratum corneum) at a healthy clip. There's a complete turnover of cells every 28 days. The hormonal turmoil of the teens is easing, and oil glands are no longer overstimulated, which is the major cause of acne.

On the other hand, a cyclical stream of the hormones estrogen and progesterone keeps just enough oil flowing to maintain a natural moisture balance. A cushion of fat above the facial muscles pads the bony architecture, softens angles, and plumps the hollows, while the protein fibers elastin and collagen give the skin resilience and toughness. Twentysomething skin has moisture, good circulation, and bounce.

Fighting back: Some women may continue to experience premenstrual breakouts when progesterone surges and activates oil glands or when stress triggers a release of the hormone. When drying or antibiotic lotions aren't enough, oral antibiotics—or oral contraceptives—can help. (Accutane, the brand name for isotretinoin, may be prescribed for serious adult acne. But because of the risk of birth defects, the drug is only for women who are committed to practicing birth control.) The sun protection used now determines how youthful skin will remain. A UVA- and UVB-blocking sunscreen and wraparound sunglasses help prevent wrinkles. And women who smoke should stop. That causes wrinkles, too.

Thirties: A More Pragmatic View of Beauty

In our thirties, life may become more complicated. But at least our identities—and, therefore, our attitudes toward our appearances—are more clear-cut.

"The thirties bring so much more freedom about self-image," says Dr. Johnston. "We're working, and we're mothers, and we think, 'Beauty is one part of who I am, but not all of who I am.' It's less critical to our self-esteem."

Logically, makeup and skin care become less a form of identification and more a routine. "Rather than constantly striving to be a certain way and never being happy, I think 'How much effort do I want to put into this?'" says Dr. Johnston. "It's a more peaceful, rational approach."

And more practical. "You should cut down on certain regimens and go for the sure things," advises makeup artist Pablo Manzoni. "In beauty, this means a worry-free haircut and around-the-clock moisturizing."

This doesn't necessarily translate into boring, though. "At 30, women who have experimented have calmed down a bit and learned what makes them look best," says Nars. "But they're still open to trying new things."

Greenwell calls these years the enhancement period. "You've cultivated a look, but everything gets softer and better applied," she says. "You're still fashionable, but you're making the best of yourself."

Although they're feeling more secure about their strengths, both internal and external, women in their thirties are starting to worry about looking older. They suddenly see a laugh line, a frown line, crow's-feet, gray hairs—every woman has a moment of reckoning. Let's hope she's too busy to dwell on it.

Your skin: This period could be considered the calm before the storm. Damage from time and sun is accumulating but is not yet visible. Collagen fibers are being lost at a rate of about 1 percent per year, and the ones that remain are beginning to go slack. Sunlight accelerates the loss. It also damages the tiny capillaries that provide the skin with a nourishing blood supply. As a result, grooves form between the brows, laugh lines appear around the corners of the eyes, and the folds from the corner of the nose to the mouth begin to deepen.

Fighting back: Cell turnover is slowing, and dead cells that clump on the skin's surface dull the complexion. Exfoliation with scrubs or alpha hydroxy acid creams removes dry cells and boosts cell turnover. Topical antioxidants may help destroy DNA-damaging, wrinkle-enhancing chemicals that are created when the sun hits the skin.

Forties: Update Your Beauty Routine

In the years leading up to menopause, a woman can expect a number of inevitable physical changes. Her skin becomes drier, and her metabolism slows down. More fat is stored in her hips and thighs. If she doesn't exercise regularly, her muscle tone diminishes. Her hair may become gray and listless. And the lines in her face, which seemed charming at age 35, are now more pronounced and more annoying—and more in number.

The good news is that women are taking better care of themselves today than ever before. "I don't see much difference between women in their thirties and forties these days," says Nars. "I don't know if it's diet, exercise, or surgery, but it's happening."

Still, women may realize they've lost something that they once took for granted, whether it's a smooth forehead or a firm jawline. "The forties can be unstable years," says Reiss-Andersen. "But that's when you start searching for real solutions (in skin care and cosmetics), not just routines."

By the time women reach their forties, "they are very careful about diet and exercise, and they drink less alcohol," says Manzoni, whose clientele is mostly over 40. "They're doing masks and getting peels, and they're intensely lubricating their skin. Careful skin care and extremely accurate makeup are the marks of a classic 40-year-old. She is accomplished. She has arrived."

Psychologists make the same observation. "People say we live in a cult of youth, but I don't agree," says New York City psychologist Sheenah Hankin. "The older you get, the more power you get."

Based on what she has seen in her clinical work, Dr. Johnston looks forward to her forties. "In many women, I see a certain confidence emerge. They develop their own style."

Along those lines, Dr. Then advises clients in their forties to update their looks with new makeup colors and to get rid of the gray. "What you think about your looks is as important as what you actually look like," she says.

Women have other ways to look gorgeous despite gravity's pull, such as using liquid foundation during the day and a rich moisturizer at night and trying new makeup techniques. "You can't use the same tricks as before," says Greenwell. "If you love wearing eyeliner and the sides of your eyes have begun to droop, it won't look as good." Instead, focus on lifting and restructuring features. "A wonderful trick is to stroke eye shadow up and out, not down," she suggests. "It actually makes the eyes look lifted." And to illuminate the face, Greenwell is a big believer in blush. "By the time you're in your forties, you know the best place to apply it. You understand your face."

At this time in your life, it's important not to get stuck in a rut. Reiss-Andersen's solution: Check out other people with similar looks and coloring to see what they're doing. Go to department stores and scout out the hipper counters. This doesn't mean your beauty routine has to get complicated, stresses Reiss-Andersen—just more contemporary. "It could mean using lengthening mascara or switching to a lighter brow pencil," she notes. "Eye shadow with a little shimmer could be a good change, as could wearing sheerer lipstick without lines." That's great advice at any age.

Your skin: Decades of wear and tear are really making their mark. The network of fine elastin fibers is being replaced by thicker, stiffer fibers. Skin sags, expression lines deepen, and areas of the face are crosshatched with fine wrinkles. Brown spots crop up on the cheeks (as well as the backs of the hands). Tiny blood vessels stretch, twist, and leak. Clusters of them may appear as spidery tendrils near the skin's surface. Those who avoided the sun in and before their twenties and thirties can now cash in on their conscientiousness, showing far less damage than those who soaked up the rays.

Fighting back: Skin, which loses some 30 percent of its water content as it ages, becomes prone to dryness. More frequent moisturizing is needed to help keep it supple and smooth. Daily use of a skin-bleaching cream can eliminate brown spots and other areas of discoloration (or hyperpigmentation). Cleansing with a gentle soap substitute maintains the skin's natural oils, while a thicker, richer moisturizer applied at night helps maximize the skin's capacity to hold water. Drinking at least eight eight-ounce glasses of water, herbal tea, and juice a day helps.

Creases that come from sleeping with your head in the same position all night may now last well into the day. Sleeping on a down pillow with a satin cover will minimize wrinkles.

Fifties: Attitude Is Everything

Beauty in the fifties depends very much on the individual, more so than during other decades. "Some women still look young and try to maintain that," points out Reiss-Andersen. "Others determine that they are classics and go for a foolproof look that has very little to do with fashion. They wear classic red lipstick, for example—something that will give them the ladies-who-lunch look they are entitled to at that age." The worst thing a 50-year-old woman can do, adds Reiss-Andersen, is try to look 20.

Psychologically, the fifties can be a bit more complex. "When my mother was 56, she was attractive but had given up on beauty," notes Hankin. "I'm 56, and I haven't given up at all. Self-preservation is great. I find myself becoming a lot more interested in skin products. It's much more fun to battle age and stay sexy as you get older, because you're more comfortable."

On the other hand, observes Dr. Then, "I hear women saying all the time that they start to feel socially invisible in their fifties. This is true even of women who take really good care of themselves, wear expensive clothes, and have well-groomed hair and nails." Why are they ignored? "They're just no longer 25," she says.

This harsh reality, she notes, is exactly what propels so many women to the plastic surgeon's office. She wishes women would focus on the big picture instead. "Looking good and feeling healthy and happy—that's what women should go for now," advises Dr. Then. "Know what looks good on you and what doesn't." If your arms aren't tight, don't wear sleeveless shirts. Conversely, if your legs are toned, wear skirts that stop above the knees.

And if wrinkles around your eyes are a sore spot, enhance your lashes and brows instead. "Make the eyes more vivid with mascara, and skip the rest," suggests Reiss-Andersen. "Or do something subtle with shadow. Skip the whole elaborate technique."

Your skin: The face is now mature. The fat padding beneath the skin has diminished, so unless a woman experiences significant weight gain, her face shows more of its angles and hollows. As muscle fibers slacken, the fat that remains under the eyes forms bags. Facial bones begin to shrink, particularly in smokers, causing all-around sagging.

Skin-cell turnover slows, and collagen and elastin fibers break down. In sun-damaged skin, the uppermost layers thicken and the pores enlarge. In skin that has been protected, these layers become thin and flat. Gravity continues to take its toll on the eyelids, nose, and ears, and the upper lip thins. Overall, genes and sun exposure determine how radically a woman's face ages.

Fighting back: After menopause, the oil glands start to give out. Rich moisturizers containing alpha hydroxy acids or lactic acid can help, as can avoiding harsh toners and astringents. Hormone replacement therapy after menopause preserves skin elasticity and prevents dryness and bone loss. (Taking progesterone in addition to estrogen is believed to be less likely to cause uterine cancer. But women with strong family histories of breast cancer are still at risk for that disease.)

40

Fast Fixes for Tired Eyes

The eyes are a window on the human soul. They express moods and emotions that sometimes even words cannot.

Unfortunately, they also announce to the world when you've had a late night out. Or a lousy night's sleep. Or a good bawl at the end of your favorite romantic flick.

Dark circles and puffy eyes certainly cloud an otherwise radiant face. Throw in those tiny lines known as crow's-feet, and one glance in the mirror can leave you feeling old before your time.

The good news is that you can make these eye-noyances vanish—or, in the case of crow's-feet, prevent them from occurring in the first place. Here's how.

Look Refreshed in a Flash

You can make dark circles and puffy eyes fade fast. Just follow this simple morning-after routine recommended by Trisha Sawyer, makeup artist for actresses Geena Davis and Sharon Stone.

The first thing you want to do, before putting on even a drop of makeup, is depuff and smooth your skin. This prevents your makeup from settling and cracking, creating a caked-on look. Gently wash your face, then apply a skin-tightening moisturizer around your eyes. (Look for one in your favorite skin-care line, or try Eye Specialists or Uplift by Prescriptives.)

Crow's-Feet Take a Hike

Plastic surgeons have discovered a substance that can make crow's-feet disappear in a matter of days. What is this anti-aging tonic? Botulinum toxin—the same substance that causes botulism, a serious and potentially fatal form of food poisoning.

Doctors have been using botulinum toxin, which is produced by the bacterium *Clostridium botulinum*, since the 1970s to treat a variety of conditions affecting facial nerves and muscles. More recently, botulinum toxin injections have been used by aesthetic plastic surgeons to erase crow's-feet, frown lines, forehead furrows, and wrinkles of the lower face.

Some lines and wrinkles result from facial muscles that overcontract when you frown or squint. Botulinum toxin works by blocking the transmission of impulses from nerve cells to the facial muscles. This interferes with the muscles' ability to contract.

"If you can freeze the muscle, you can stop a wrinkle," explains Alan Matarasso, M.D., associate professor of plastic surgery at Albert Einstein College of Medicine in New York City.

"I'm very excited about botulinum toxin injections because they allow plastic surgeons to target the facial muscles that cause wrinkles, not just treat the wrinkles themselves," says Dr. Matarasso. "The injections require no surgery or general anesthesia. It's a fast, simple, safe in-office procedure."

The effects of the treatment usually last from one to five months, so it must be repeated periodically. So far, plastic surgeons who administer botulinum toxin injections have noted some temporary side effects: a burning sensation during injection; local numbness, swelling, or bruising; headaches or nausea; and mild to moderate drooping of one or both eyelids.

Botulinum toxin injections shouldn't be administered to pregnant or lactating women, says Dr. Matarasso. Doctors don't yet know whether the toxin can harm a developing fetus or a nursing infant. The injections also are not appropriate for women taking certain types of antibiotics.

To find a plastic surgeon trained to administer botulinum toxin injections, call the American Society for Aesthetic Plastic Surgery. Check toll-free directory assistance for the number.

HEALTH FLASH

Next, settle down for two to five minutes with a chilled, steeped chamomile or green tea bag over each eye. The natural properties of these herbal teas help bring puffy eyes back down to size. While you wait, breathe deeply and try to relax. Then remove the tea bags and apply your foundation as usual—no need to rinse first.

When touching up dark under-eye circles, be sure to apply your concealer low on the eye sockets, not under your bottom lashes. Be careful not to cover any puffy areas. "Concealer has a light-reflective quality that only accentuates the swelling," Sawyer explains.

Adding color to the rest of your face can help de-emphasize your eyes. If your skin seems pale, Sawyer suggests brightening it up with a dusting of blush on the apples of your cheeks. She also recommends using rosy lipsticks rather than darker ones, to create a more refreshed look.

Head Off Crow's-Feet

Unlike puffy eyes and dark circles, crow's-feet don't appear overnight. Nor will they disappear—at least not without the aid of peels, injections, or surgery.

So what can you do to slow the appearance of those telltale wrinkles at the corners of your eyes? "Start the prevention process now," recommends Seth L. Matarasso, M.D., associate clinical professor of dermatology at the University of California, San Francisco, School of Medicine. Practice the following good habits while crow's-feet are still fine lines, and you should be able to keep smiling—wrinkle-free—a lot longer.

Safeguard against the sun. Who hasn't heard that Old Sol is the skin's greatest enemy? As if the ultraviolet rays themselves weren't bad enough, squinting to shield your eyes from bright light also exacerbates wrinkle formation. Wear a sunscreen with a sun protection factor (SPF) of 15 or greater every day. Also invest in Jackie O–type sunglasses or, even better, wraparounds.

Roll over. If you sleep on your side or stomach, try switching to your back instead. "Sleeping on the same side every night essentially presses the same wrinkles into your face," Dr. Matarasso explains. Sleeping on your back helps smooth out the wrinkles because gravity works to pull the skin backward. If you find that you absolutely cannot sleep on your back, at least try to switch sides frequently.

Handle with care. The skin below your eyes is thin and has few oil-producing glands. So don't pull, tug, or drag it as you apply and remove makeup. Any time you apply cream or lotion, dab, don't rub. Choose smooth-gliding eye makeup—a soft eyeliner pencil rather than a hard one, for example. And allow makeup remover to set for an extra 30 seconds before wiping it off. That way, the product—not your rubbing motion—does the removing.

Quick Fix for Puffy Lids

Don't have any chamomile or green tea bags on hand? One of the fastest, easiest, and cheapest ways to reduce puffiness around your eyes is with a glass of ice water and four stainless steel spoons, says Seth L. Matarasso, M.D., associate clinical professor of dermatology at the University of California, San Francisco, School of Medicine. Chill the spoons in the water, then place one over each eye. When the spoons become warm, switch them with the others chilling in the glass of water. Keep switching until you see improvement.

Investigate Retin-A. Dr. Matarasso has found that prolonged regular use of Retin-A cream, an acne product that exfoliates the skin, also improves the appearance of fine crow's-feet. He prefers Retin-A to Renova, a similar product designed specifically for wrinkles, because the former is available in a lower concentration. This is important, because using too strong a formulation of either Retin-A or Renova can cause redness, swelling, and scaling of the skin. Since Retin-A is a prescription product, you'll need to consult a dermatologist if you wish to try it.

Note: Sunscreen protection is absolutely essential for anyone using Retin-A or Renova.

Fuss-Free Care for Fabulous Hair

D irk swept Vanessa into his arms. She saw in his eyes a love that she had never known before, had never dreamed possible. And as he softly stroked her fine, limp hair . . ."

Wait a minute—that can't be! Everybody knows that the heroes and heroines of dime-store romance novels have lustrous, luxurious manes. You know the kind: There's no peril great enough—not facing down a band of bad guys, standing in the path of a speeding locomotive, or hanging by a fingertip from a 100-foot cliff—to undo these indestructible 'dos.

We mere mortals, of course, have to deal with more everyday stresses to our tresses. Even the process of caring for our hair—the washing, drying, and styling—does its share of damage. A combination of the right cleansing and styling products and good grooming techniques can help ensure that your hair always looks and feels its healthiest.

Picking the Right Products

Perhaps the most important part of your hair-care regimen is deciding which shampoo and conditioner to use. Heaven knows, there are plenty to choose from. When shopping around, keep these tips in mind.

Let your hide be your guide. Your scalp should determine which cleansing product you use, advises Philip Kingsley, owner of Philip Kingsley Trichological (hair and scalp) Centres in New York City and London. If it tends to be dry, for example, use a mild shampoo as well as a conditioner.

If it's very dry, try this homemade treatment recommended by Diana Bihova, M.D., clinical assistant professor of dermatology at New York University Medical Center in New York City: Mix a little bath oil with water and apply it to your scalp. Wrap your head with a towel, turban-style, then wait for one hour before shampooing.

Try before you buy. What about shampoos formulated for special needs, such as fine or processed hair? You can't necessarily go by the label, since everyone's hair responds to such products differently. Your best bet, Dr. Bihova says, is to audition shampoos. Buy sample sizes and try them until you find one that you like.

Trade off occasionally. If you're using a deep-conditioning shampoo, switch to a deep-cleaning formula—designed to remove buildup—at least once a week, says Rebecca J. Caserio, M.D., clinical associate professor of dermatology at the University of Pittsburgh. "Oftentimes the conditioning agents in certain shampoos—as well as the calcium, magnesium, and iron salts in hard water—cause buildup on the hair shaft," she explains. Removing this buildup restores bounce and fullness to hair that has become lifeless and flat.

Get into condition. A conditioner can add moisture, nutrients, and shine to your hair. As with shampoos, there are many different conditioning products to choose from, each one targeting a specific hair type. Go with a lighter conditioner if you have fine, thin hair and a heavier conditioner if you have coarse or curly hair, Kingsley advises.

For damaged or chemically treated hair, also apply a deep conditioner once or twice a week. Some deep-conditioning products are applied before shampooing, allowed to set, and then washed out. Others are leave-ins, meaning that you work them into your hair after it has been shampooed but while it's still wet. As for how much deep conditioner you should use, that's a matter of trial and error, Kingsley says.

Common Hair-Care Mistakes

Just because you've been shampooing since you were a little kid doesn't mean that you're doing it right. Yes, there is a best way to wash and dry your hair, according to Kingsley. Using the proper techniques may not solve all of your hair woes, but it will ensure better-looking, healthier hair in the long run.

Here are the common mistakes most people make—and how to fix them.

Not detangling first. Before you even wet your hair, run a wide-toothed comb through it to remove tangles.

Using your fingernails to shampoo. Your nails may damage your scalp or make it bleed. Instead, gently massage your scalp with your fingertips. Continue the massaging action for about three minutes.

Rinsing too quickly. A good rinsing to remove all of the shampoo takes longer than most people suspect. When you think you've rinsed enough, rinse again. If you don't wash your hair daily, repeat the shampoo and rinse process twice, making the second rinse a good, long one.

Rubbing conditioner into the roots. Apply conditioner over your rinsed hair, particularly to the ends. Do not rub it into your scalp or put it on the hair roots. Conditioner is for the hair, not the scalp. The damaged ends need it most.

Leaving conditioner on too long. Rinse out conditioner immediately unless it is meant to be applied as a treatment before shampooing. Leaving it in too long can cause your hair to become dull.

Detangling from the roots. After towel-drying your hair, ease out any tangles with a wide-toothed comb. Start at the ends and work your way toward your scalp in short segments. Starting from the top means that you're bunching the tangles together. The tugging needed to remove them could damage your hair.

Wash Away Tension

A shampoo is a perfect time to treat yourself to a gentle, relaxing head massage. "It's nurturing," says Meg Waldron, a neuromuscular massage therapist in Bernardsville, New Jersey. "Your body knows you're taking care of yourself."

The next time you lather up your locks, follow these four steps.

1. With your thumbs at the nape of your neck, make circular motions. Slowly work your way up to the crown of your head.
2. Gently press your fingertips into the sides of your head, just above your ears. Using small circular and up-and-down movements, work your way to the top of your head and then to the front.
3. Move your fingertips in large circles over your entire scalp.
4. Lightly massage your temples, again using circular motions with your fingertips. Apply gentle pressure. Brisk scrubbing can break wet hair, Waldron notes.

In addition to the personal pampering and relaxation benefits, massaging your head during a shampoo increases circulation in the scalp, helps remove dry skin, and provides a deep cleansing effect.

Apply Makeup Like a Pro

Remember the good old days at the drugstore makeup counter, when you and your friends invested your babysitting earnings in bright orange lipstick, green mascara, and frosted eye shadow in four shades of pastel?

Ouch. If you were to try pulling that off today, chances are someone would ask how much you would charge to be the clown at her kid's birthday party.

To be sure, some makeup techniques that you've used for years may make you appear older than you are. But the right cosmetics, properly applied, can help you maintain a look that's young, fresh, and full of life.

Putting Your Best Face Forward

Cosmetologists and other makeup pros have developed scores of clever techniques for helping women use cosmetics to their advantage. Here are their top 10 tricks of the trade.

Head in the right direction. Always blend foundation in whichever direction the tiny hairs on your face grow. This keeps the hairs from "ruffing up" and makes the surface of your skin look smooth.

Use a light hand. When you're applying under-eye concealer, remember that less is more. A too-heavy layer can cake, making bags and circles more obvious.

Make eye makeup last. If you wear powdered eye shadow, apply concealer to your eyelids first. This helps keep the eye shadow in place.

Makeup for Problem Skin

In the long run, acne-fighting lotion keeps you looking great. But under makeup, it creates a chalky, uneven appearance and can even throw off the colors.

Enter a new acne lotion with a glycerin base. In a recent study of 50 women, two-thirds who tried this glycerin-based benzoyl peroxide product (brand name Triaz) preferred it to a similar product with a water base (Benzamycin). Since both contain benzoyl peroxide—a common prescription and over-the-counter acne treatment—they have equal acne-fighting power, says the study's author, Zoe Draelos, M.D., clinical associate professor in the department of dermatology at Bowman Gray University School of Medicine in Winston-Salem, North Carolina. What's more, the glycerin base is more moisturizing than water, hence the great all-day look.

Currently, Triaz is the only glycerin-based benzoyl peroxide product on the market. It's available by prescription.

Try color in threes. To give your eyes a simple yet polished look, choose three similar shades of eye shadow, from light to dark. Apply the light shade all over your lid. Follow with the medium shade along the crease on your eyelid or just on the lower lid. Finish with the dark shade just above the lash line.

Pump up the volume. Dot black pencil eyeliner between your eyelashes, upper and lower. This makes your lashes appear fuller without mascara.

Extend the life of eyeliner. To make eyeliner last longer, apply a powder liner or an eye shadow close to the last line, using an eyeliner brush dipped in water. If you use a pencil liner, set it with translucent powder afterward.

Come together at the corner. Make sure that the eyeliner on the top and bottom of your eye meets at the outer corner. Otherwise, your eye looks shortened and unnatural.

Play down circles. If you have a problem with under-eye circles, don't apply eyeliner or mascara underneath your eyes. It casts a dark shadow, emphasizing the circles.

Stay within the lines. When applying blush, keep in mind that it should never extend farther forward than your pupil or lower than the tip of your nose.

Prolong the life of lipstick. To make lip color last, apply it like nail polish. Begin with a base coat of lip balm, followed by two color coats—lip liner and lipstick. Finish up with a topcoat of translucent powder (dusted onto your lips through one ply of tissue).

Face the Facts about Face-Lifts

Listen in on any group of women over age 40, and you may hear the conversation eventually turn to cosmetic surgery. Face-lifts. Brow lifts. Eyelid-lifts. Laser peels. Who has had what? Who wants what?

In 1996, 3,204,430 Americans had cosmetic surgery—enough people to fill the city of Miami and most of Fort Lauderdale. No one is keeping track of the dollars spent on cosmetic improvements. But three-million-plus people at $1,000 to $7,000 a pop isn't pocket change.

Still, for every woman who makes the decision to go under the knife, so to speak, many more are just beginning to traverse the rocky emotional terrain of cosmetic surgery. "Am I really the kind of person who would cave in to the social pressure to look young?" they wonder. "Why can't I just age gracefully?"

In this chapter, other smart, honest women share how they decided for or against cosmetic surgery and what getting it—or not getting it—was like. Their stories may help you decide if a face-lift is in your future.

Pat: "My Face Had Collapsed"

Pat Arnold had her first face-lift in the early 1960s. She was 38, a smoker, and a sun-worshiper. "What I saw in the mirror was that my face had collapsed. I looked 55. I was too young to look so old."

Pat was a commercial pilot, forging a new career for a woman. "I didn't want to look like an old lady flying a plane." Not only that, "I used to be good-looking, and I was accustomed to being admired. I started to drink to put it out of my mind."

When she scheduled surgery, "I was so excited. Even if I died, it would be worth it." She did almost die. She went into shock after excess blood loss. "But I looked so good after the face-lift, I had something done every four or five years. I probably overdid it. I'd tell people that I had been in an auto accident to explain the bruises. There wasn't a lot of pain, except for the chemical peel. That was like a third-degree burn—almost unbearable. But worth it. I had baby-soft skin."

Her last lift was more than 10 years ago. "Now I accept the way I look. But back then, surgery saved me from giving up on life."

Sara: "My Husband Thought Cosmetic Surgery Was Terrible"

When she was 50, Sara Cohn had eyelid surgery to remove the "genetic" puffiness around her eyes. "I hated the way they looked. Makeup would get stuck in the folds.

"I didn't do any soul-searching about it. But my husband thought it was terrible. He was afraid something would go wrong and wreck our happiness."

Despite that, he nursed her through the first hours after surgery. "A day later, I was up and out," she says. "One thing was a problem, though. My eyes were so tight in the beginning that I couldn't shut them. I was worried about it, but it eased up."

Today, Sara is planning another face-lift. And that has required a lot of soul-searching. "My husband can't even talk about it. Lots of things could go wrong. I questioned myself: What price vanity? But my desire has overcome all that. I want to feel better when I look in the mirror. I've never heard anyone say that she was sorry she did it."

Patsy: "Your Age Becomes This Ugly Secret"

Patricia McLaughlin is a syndicated fashion columnist. She regularly attends New York City fashion shows. But she won't completely cover her gray hair, much less schedule cosmetic surgery.

"I would do anything to be prettier, unless it's hard or painful or really expensive. But I'm totally suspicious of doing anything to look younger. Your age becomes this ugly secret. I don't want to live like that.

"But I have been tempted to consider surgery, like when I look in the mirror and see someone who doesn't look enough like me. It's disorienting. Most of the time, I feel that's just an indication of how screwy my values are. Pay thousands of dollars to smooth out my forehead when people are starving? Even more than that, though, it would mean admitting I'm ashamed of how I look, which means I'm ashamed of being the age I am. Even if I feel that, I can't agree with it. It's too sick."

Brenda: "This Is Just One More Thing"

A photo of herself in profile sent Brenda Gilson to the cosmetic surgeon's office. "I saw the turkey flesh . . . I remembered how my mother's whole chin had fallen."

So Gilson got rid of what surgeons call redundant flesh. "It does hurt. I felt like I had been in a car accident. My face was kind of swollen and numb for a week. But I had it done on a Wednesday and was back at work on Monday.

"I didn't wrestle with the decision at all. I'm very vain. I don't think there's anything to be gained spiritually from wrestling. And I was pleased with the change. I'll go back and have more surgery when I need it. All my life I've been doing things to look good. This is just one more thing.

"I am very sensitive about having the surgery, though. I don't want it even whispered among my friends. I'm telling you only because I think it's liberating for women to hear."

Maureen: "I Want to Even the Playing Field"

Maureen O'Neil is a beautiful woman. But she doesn't agree. She's on TV, and the beauty standards are different.

"I want to even the playing field," O'Neil says. "I see people who are in their late fifties. They've had lifts, and they look great. That seems so unfair.

"I'm shocked I feel this way. I remember that when I was 33, I thought age was beautiful. Not long ago, though, I realized how unhappy I am about my face. I fought it with pep talks about inner beauty and good sense. It didn't work. I'm tired of wasting emotional energy worrying about how bad I look. I want to cross that off my list and free up that energy to live.

"In this day and age, I know I can change things. So I'm going to do it. Never before has there been a culture so emphatic about appearance. But I worry about creating a new 'should'—'you should be thin'—and creating a chasm between those women who can afford it and those who can't."

How about You?

Like the women described above, you may have your own reasons for contemplating cosmetic surgery. Only you can know for certain whether it's appropriate for you. In terms of altering your appearance, it's a much more drastic measure than, say, changing your hairstyle.

And it is an ordeal. "You really have to have your mind on it, not on anything else," says Craig Foster, M.D., a plastic surgeon in New York City. "You shouldn't do it if you're having trouble at work or in your marriage or with your kids. You have to get your life settled first. You want the conditions to be as ideal as they can be for elective surgery."

Still, serious problems are rare. The most common—bumps of blood under the skin called hematomas and scars that are too big—can usually be fixed. Postoperative bruising lasts anywhere from three to six weeks.

To assess whether you're a good candidate for cosmetic surgery, take this short quiz developed by Stacey Tantleff Dunn, Ph.D., and Allison Kanter of the Laboratory for the Study of Eating, Appearance, and Health at the University of Central Florida in Orlando. Simply answer each question yes or no.

1. Have I spent a great deal of time weighing the costs (emotional, physical, financial) and benefits of having this surgery?
2. Am I fully informed of the physical risks involved in undergoing surgery?

Turn Back the Clock without Surgery

Before you plunk down a bundle of money for cosmetic surgery, try these self-care strategies. They'll help erase signs of aging and restore youthful vitality to your appearance.

❖ Wear sunscreen daily. "Most people don't realize that regular use of sunscreen can actually reverse mild damage caused by the sun," says Joshua Wieder, M.D., assistant clinical professor at the University of California, Los Angeles.

❖ In addition to sunscreen, apply a glycolic (alpha hydroxy) or salicyclic (beta hydroxy) acid product every morning. It decreases surface roughness, the appearance of fine lines, and brown spots, Dr. Wieder says.

❖ Avoid direct sunlight, tanning parlors, and reflective surfaces such as snow and water. And remember that certain antibiotics can make you extra-sensitive to the sun.

❖ Sleep on your back. Temporary lines and creases develop when your face is pressed directly into your pillow, especially if you sleep on the same side each night.

❖ Stop smoking. Smoke breaks down collagen, leading to fine lines, and makes skin sallow. And the act of drawing in smoke creates wrinkles around the lips.

❖ Guard your face against extreme temperatures by wearing a heavy moisturizer in cold weather.

❖ If you're prone to broken capillaries, avoid anything that will make your face redden, such as saunas, hot drinks, alcoholic beverages, and spicy foods.

❖ Avoid manipulating the delicate skin around your eyes. The more you stretch it, the less elasticity it will retain. Use a good eye makeup remover and a soft cotton pad, so you don't have to rub hard. And if you wear contact lenses, try to put in your lenses and drops without excessively tugging on your skin.

❖ Eat garlic. Researchers discovered that human cell cultures survived longer and kept a more "youthful" appearance when garlic was added.

❖ Drink lots of water, get eight hours of sleep each night, and use a moisturizer daily to keep your skin hydrated, radiant, and soft.

3. Do I understand all of the medical information that I have received?
4. Do I expect that having this surgery will significantly change my life?
5. Is someone else (spouse, friend, relative) persuading me to have this surgery?
6. Do most people tell me this surgery is unnecessary or seem unable to understand why I am dissatisfied with my appearance?

7. Do I expect my doctor to tell me what change(s) will make me look best?
8. Have I recently experienced a stressful event or crisis in my life (such as the death of a loved one or divorce)?
9. Have I been experiencing psychological or emotional problems such as depression, anxiety, or an eating disorder?
10. Do I believe that having this surgery will really please others who are important to me?

If you responded no to questions 1, 2, or 3, or if you responded yes to any of the remaining questions, you may want to seriously reevaluate your decision to have cosmetic surgery. Counseling by a licensed therapist, preferably one knowledgeable about body image, may help you further explore your options and make a well-informed decision.

Choosing a Surgeon

If you decide to go ahead with cosmetic surgery, your first and most important step is picking the proper professional to do it. Plastic surgeons are trained in invasive procedures such as face-lifts, brow-lifts, and eye-lifts. Dermatological surgeons work on the surface of the skin, burning or sanding away fine lines and wrinkles. But they also do cosmetic surgery, as do otolaryngologists (ear, nose, and throat specialists) and opthalmologists.

Before you choose, schedule consultations with two or three doctors. Be aware, though, that all three may have diverging opinions. Usually, the difference comes down to aesthetic judgment or which procedure each is most comfortable performing. Do be leery if a doctor says you need a grocery list of procedures when you just want one or two.

The following tips can also help you find the right surgeon for the job.

❖ Get recommendations from your relatives and friends— preferably those who have had the procedure you want.
❖ Check whether the specialist you choose is board-certified in that specialty.
❖ Make sure that the doctor is affiliated with a hospital, even if she performs the operations in her office or an ambulatory center. It's a sign of quality control.
❖ If the surgeon operates in her office, make sure the operating room has been approved by the American Association for Accreditation of Ambulatory Surgery Facilities. Ask if she has emergency resuscitation and postoperative monitoring equipment readily available.
❖ Make sure the doctor is licensed by calling the medical surveillance office of your local government. Ask if any complaints or violations have been filed against that doctor.

❖ Find out which court handles lawsuits in the same jurisdiction as your prospective surgeon's office. Then check whether any suits have been filed against her.

❖ Ask about the training of the doctor and her staff. If she performs laser surgery, find out how she learned. Look for someone who has done a preceptorship—a course in which doctors work alongside a skilled laser specialist over a period of time.

❖ Ask the surgeon how long she has been performing the procedure you want. Ask how many times she has done it in the past six months. There is no "magic" number to listen for, but generally, surgeons who work at a laser center or who have more than one laser system have a good amount of laser experience.

If a doctor seems angered by your questions or reluctant to answer them, take that as your cue to move on. On the other hand, if all of the doctors you consult pass your test with flying colors, choose the one you're most comfortable with. That's most likely the person who answered all of your questions without rushing, gave you all the information you wanted about pre- and post-op care, and explained your procedure in full.

Credits

"Overhaul Your Medicine Cabinet" on page 19 is adapted from "What Every Medicine Cabinet Needs," an article by Catherine Houck that originally appeared in *New Woman*. Copyright © 1998 by Catherine Houck. Reprinted with permission.

"Hormone Replacement Update" on page 26 is adapted from "A Safer Estrogen," an article by Rosie Mestel that originally appeared in *Health*. Copyright © 1997 by *Health*. Reprinted with permission.

"Long Live Older Mothers" on page 27 is adapted from an article of the same name that originally appeared in *Health*. Copyright © 1997 by *Health*. Reprinted with permission.

"When Menopause Won't Wait" on page 33 is adapted from "Early Menopause," an article by Sarah Schafer that originally appeared in *Self*. Copyright © 1997 by the Condé Nast Publications, Inc. Courtesy *Self*.

"How Healthy Is Your Family Tree?" on page 44 is adapted from "Are You at Risk? 10 Questions You Must Ask Your Mom," an article by Erica Lumière that originally appeared in *Family Circle*. Copyright © 1998 by Gruner + Jahr USA Publishing. Reprinted with permission of *Family Circle* magazine.

"Breakthroughs in Breast Health" on page 47 contains text adapted from "Erase Exam Anxiety," an article by Megan Othersen Gorman that originally appeared in *Prevention's Guide to Fit and Firm at 40 Plus*. Copyright © 1998 by Megan Othersen Gorman. Reprinted with permission.

"The Latest Strategies for Stronger Bones" on page 64 is adapted from "Age-proof Your Body," an article by Gayle Feldman that originally appeared in *New Woman*. Copyright © 1998 by Gayle Feldman. Reprinted with permission.

"Help for an Aching Head" on page 82 is adapted from "Headache Healing," an article by Chris Bohjalian that originally appeared in *New Woman*. Copyright © 1998 by Chris Bohjalian. Reprinted by permission of the author.

"Help Yourself to More Sleep" on page 93 is adapted from "The Rest of Your Life," an article by James Sturz that originally appeared in *Prevention's Guide to Fit and Firm at 40 Plus*. Copyright © 1998 by James Sturz. Reprinted with permission.

"Get Up Earlier on the Weekends" on page 96 is adapted from "Tired? Get Up Earlier on Weekends," an article that originally appeared in *Heart & Soul*. Copyright © 1998 by B.E.T. Publications. Reprinted with permission.

"Supercharge Your Energy Now" on page 98 is adapted from "What Science Knows about Boosting Your Energy," an article by Allison Kornet that originally appeared in *New Woman*. Copyright © 1997 by Allison Kornet. Reprinted with permission.

"The Most Common Weight-Loss Questions Answered" on page 112 is adapted from "21 Diet Questions," an article by Susan Goodman that originally appeared in *Prevention*. Copyright © 1998 by Susan Goodman. Reprinted with permission.

"Why You Should Sniff Before You Eat" on page 119 is adapted from "Why You Should Smell Before You Eat," an article that originally appeared in *Heart & Soul*. Copyright © 1998 by B.E.T. Publications. Reprinted with permission.

"Be Fruitful and Subtract Pounds" on page 129 is adapted from "A Fruitful Diet Aid?" an article that originally appeared in *Health*. Copyright © 1998 by *Health*. Reprinted with permission.

"Do I Have to Exercise?" on page 134 is adapted from "How Hard Do You Really Need to Exercise?" an article by Nancy Monson that originally appeared in *Prevention's Guide to Total Fitness*. Copyright © 1997 by Nancy Monson. Reprinted with permission.

"No-Sweat Ways to Burn Calories All Day" on page 139 is adapted from "75 Fitness Quickies," an article by Ruth Houston that originally appeared in *Heart & Soul*. Copyright © 1998 by B.E.T. Publications. Reprinted with permission.

"Stop Feeding Your Emotions" on page 170 is adapted from "Are You Swallowing Your Emotions?" an article by Densie Webb, Ph.D., that originally appeared in *Heart & Soul*. Copyright © 1998 by B.E.T. Publications. Reprinted with permission.

"Smart Picks in the Supermarket" on page 188 is adapted from "Food Face-Off," an article by Liz Applegate, Ph.D., that originally appeared in *Runner's World*. Copyright © 1997 by Liz Applegate. Reprinted with permission.

"Margarine: Down for the Count?" on page 189 is adapted from "Stick Margarine Takes Another Hit," an article that originally appeared in *Health*. Copyright © 1997 by *Health*. Reprinted with permission.

"Where Do You Stand on the Stress Scale?" on page 214 is adapted from "How Stressed Are You?" an article that originally appeared in *First for Women*. Copyright © 1997 by Bauer Publishing Company. Reprinted with permission.

"Prescriptions for Total Serenity" on page 216 is adapted from "Top Priorities: Five Lifesaving Prescriptions for Your Mind, Body, and Soul," an article by Mariah Yeager that originally appeared in *Fitness*. Copyright © 1998 by Selene Yeager. Reprinted with permission.

"20 Instant Stress Relievers" on page 220 contains text adapted from "12 Surefire Tension Tamers," an article that originally appeared in *Heart & Soul*. Copyright © 1998 by B.E.T. Publications. Reprinted with permission.

"Where Does the Time Go?" on page 227 is adapted from "How Americans Are Killing Time," an article that originally appeared in *Health*. Copyright © 1997 by *Health*. Reprinted with permission.

"When 'Good Enough' Is Good Enough" on page 230 is adapted from "Too Perfect for Your Own Good," an article by Debra Birnbaum that originally appeared in *New Woman*. Copyright © 1998 by Debra Birnbaum. Reprinted with permission.

"Be a Super Mom, Not Supermom" on page 236 is adapted from *The Sacrificial Mother: Escaping the Trap of Self-Denial* by Carin Rubenstein, Ph.D. Copyright © 1998 by Carin Rubenstein. Reprinted with permission of Hyperion.

"What's Your Relationship IQ?" on page 244 is adapted from "Are You Compatible?" an article by David H. Olson, Ph.D., that originally appeared in *Shape*. Copyright © 1997 by David H. Olson. Reprinted with permission of the author.

"Master Your Mate's Moods" on page 252 is adapted from "Swinging with His Moods," an article by Donna Jackson that originally appeared in *New Woman*. Copyright © 1998 by Donna Jackson. Reprinted with permission.

"Sex-Induced Amnesia" on page 258 is adapted from "Morning-After Memory Lapse," an article that originally appeared in *Health*. Copyright © 1997 by *Health*. Reprinted with permission.

"Look Your Best at Any Age" on page 266 is adapted from "From Here to Eternity," an article by Jennifer Tung that originally appeared in *Allure*. Copyright © 1998 by the Condé Nast Publications, Inc. Courtesy *Allure*.

Index

Anger, eating habits and, 171–72
Antacids, 23
Antibiotics
    for acne, 269
    digestive system and, 195
    for first-aid, 24, 25
Antihistamines
    for allergies, 19–20, 74–75
    for colds, 21
    for insect bites, 24
Antioxidants, topical, 270
Anxiety, appetite and, 172
Appendicitis, 15
Appetite. *See also* Eating habits
    anxiety and, 172
    exercise and, 160
    food smells and, 119
    pectin and, 129
    suppressants, herbal, 132
Apple juice, 190
Applesauce, 123
Aromatherapy
    crayons in, 223
    for headaches, 83, 88
    for weight loss, 119, 132–33
Arthritis, 9
    chondroitin and, 201–2
    estrogen and, 30
    glucosamine and, 201–2
Aspirin, 2, 3, 22
Astelin (Rx), 74–75
Astragalus, 41, 207
Athlete's foot, 24
ATP, energy from, 98–99, 103
Axid AR, 23
Azelastine HC1 (Rx), 74–75

B

Backaches, medications for, 22
Baths, relaxing, 97, 222
Beano, 183
Beauty
    age and, 267–72
    quiz, 264–65
Belladonna, for endometriosis, 42
Benadryl, 24, 75
Benylin Adult Formula, 21
Benzamycin, 282
Benzoyl peroxide, glycerin-based, 282

Beta-carotene
    oral contraceptives and, 187
    prescription drugs and, 130
Beta hydroxy acid creams, 287
Biceps curl, *156*
Bicycle, air, exercise, *158*
Biofeedback, for headaches, 84–85
Biological clock, energy levels and, 100
Birth control. *See* Contraceptives
Bleeding, abnormal, 36–38, 41. *See also* Menstruation
Blood pressure. *See* High blood pressure
Blood-sugar test, 17
Blue-green algae as supplement, 202
Bone density, 2, 13, 64–65, 183
    estrogen and, 26, 28, 72
    postmenopausal loss of, 28, 65
    prescription drugs and, 26, 28, 30, 31, 72
    preserving, 3, 46, 66–71
Boredom, eating habits and, 172–73
Botulinum toxin, 274
Brain function, 183
Bread, wheat vs. whole-wheat, 190
Breakfast, energy levels and, 101
Breast, weight, 115, 117
Breast cancer
    breast self-examination for detecting, 2, 3, 47–49
    DHEA and, 203
    estrogen and, 26, 29, 31, 53
    heredity and, 2, 3, 44, 51
    mammograms for detecting, 2, 3, 44, 49–51, 50
    prescription drugs and, 26, 29, 31, 48
    preventing, 44, 51, 52–54
    risk factors, 3, 51
    testing, 52, 53
    treatment, research on, 54
Breast self-examination (BSE), 2, 3, 47–49
Breathing, deep, 91, 223
Brindall berry, for appetite control, 132
Bruises, first-aid for, 25
Bryonia, for endometriosis, 41
BSE. *See* Breast self-examination
Bug bites, first-aid for, 24
Burdock, 208
    for hormonal balance, 92

Echinacea
  for colds, 76, 206
  for endometriosis, 41
Ectopic pregnancies, 14
Eczema, 24
Eggs vs. egg substitutes, 192
Electrocardiogram (EKG), 14–16
  false results from, 58
Electrolytes, exercise and, 210
Emotions. *See* Mood(s)
Endometrial ablation, 37
Endometrial cancer, 37
Endometriosis, 38–39, 39
  alternative treatment for, 41–42
Endometriosis Association, 39
Energy, personal, 98
  biological clock and, 100
  hormones and, 104–6
  increasing, 100–103
  lifestyle change and, 163
  mental, 103–4
  negative, 106
Ephedra, 131
Ergot, for heavy bleeding, 41
Estrogen. *See also* Estrogen replacement
      therapy (ERT); Hormone
      replacement therapy (HRT)
  bone density and, 65
  breast cancer and, 53
  energy levels and, 104
  fibroids and, 34
Estrogen replacement therapy (ERT), 30.
      See also Hormone replacement
      therapy (HRT)
  bone density and, 26, 28, 72
  breast cancer and, 26, 31, 72
  heart disease and, 26, 28, 63
  SERMs vs., 26–31
  uterine cancer and, 72
Eucalyptus oil, to eliminate dust mites, 75
Eucerin, 24
Evista (Rx). *See* Raloxifene
Exercise(s). *See also specific exercises*
  abdominal, 157–58
  appetite and, 160
  bone density and, 3, 66, 67–68
  breast cancer and, 52
  for busy schedules, 140–44
  colds and, 76–78
  dehydration during, 211
  depression and, 173
  diet and, 62, 160
  eating and, 115–16, 164

  energy levels and, 103, 137–38, 164
  facial, 91, 264
  headaches and, 91
  heart disease and, 60
  for home, 140–41
  increasing amount of, 168–69
  intensity of, 135–36, 137–38
  iron deficiency and, 102
  longevity and, 138
  lower body, 153–55
  making time for, 164
  mood and, 138
  for mothers, 144
  osteoporosis and, 66, 67–68
  restarting, after a break, 161
  for running errands, 142
  sex and, 262, 262
  sleep and, 97
  sports drinks and, 210, 211
  for stress relief, 221
  stretching, 148–49, 149–50
  for traveling, 142–43
  upper body, 155–57
  weight loss and, 115, 119, 120, 122,
      125, 127, 134–37
  for work, 141–42
Exercise equipment, evaluated, 146, 153
Expectorants, 21
  water as, 211
Eyes, puffy, 273–75
  cold for, 276
  tea bags for, 264, 265
Eye Specialists, 273

F

Face-lifts. *See* Cosmetic surgery
Facial steaming, 222
Family histories. *See* Hereditary health
      problems
Fasting plasma glucose (FPG) test, 9,
      17
Fat, dietary, counting grams of, 162–63
Fen-phen (Rx), 128, 129
Fertility drugs, 29
Fever
  dehydration and, 211
  ibuprofen for, 22
Feverfew, for headaches, 92
Fiber, dietary, 123, 183, 184
Fibrinogen, 28

prescription drugs and, 26, 28, 30, 31
risk factors, 59–60, 62–63
vitamin B$_6$ and, 56
Heart palpitations, 15
Heat, for headaches, 90
Heat-sensitive pads, for breast cancer detection, 53
Hemochromatosis, 16
Herbal teas, 88, 222
Herbs, medicinal, 205–8. *See also specific herbs*
for abnormal bleeding, 41
for endometriosis, 41–42
for headaches, 91–92
in snack foods, 208
for weight loss, 130–33, 133
Hereditary health problems, 44–46. *See also specific types*
HERS, 40
High blood pressure, 2–3, 60. *See also* Heart disease
diet for lowering, 7
functional foods for, 194
prescription drugs and, 129–30
sleep and, 94–95
High-density lipoprotein (HDL). *See* Cholesterol levels
Hiking trails, 151
Hormone replacement therapy (HRT), 104. *See also* Estrogen replacement therapy (ERT)
breast cancer and, 3, 31
fibroids and, 34
heart disease and, 2, 3
osteoporosis and, 3
skin health and, 267
Hormones. *See specific types*
Hot dogs, beef/pork vs. turkey, 190
Hotel stays, exercise tips for, 143
Hot flashes, prescription drugs and, 30, 31
HRT. *See* Hormone replacement therapy
Hydrocortisone cream, 24, 25
Hydrogenated vegetable oil, 189
Hypertension. *See* High blood pressure
Hyperthyroidism, 105–6
Hypofrontality, 254–55
Hypothyroidism, 105–6
Hysterectomies
for cancers, 40
for endometriosis, 38

for fibroids, 34
for heavy or abnormal bleeding, 2, 3, 36–37
unnecessary, 32
Hysterectomy Educational Resources and Services (HERS), 40

I

Ibuprofen, 3
for backaches, 22
for colds, 21
for fevers, 22
for menstrual cramps, 23
for menstrual migraines, 22
Ice, for headaches, 90
Ice cream vs. frozen yogurt, 191
Imitrex (Rx), 82
Immune system
echinacea and, 76
endometriosis and, 41
mood and, 81
vitamin E and, 77
Imodium, 23
Impaired fasting glucose, 9
Indigestion, 23
Insect bites, first-aid for, 24
Insomnia. *See also* Sleep
aspirin for, 22
melatonin for, 204
sleep position and, 95
Intelligent Cuisine, 194
IOD, 16
Iron
calcium and, 71
deficiency, 102–3, 182
in hamburgers, 192
Iron overload disease (IOD), 16
Isotretinoin (Rx), 269
Itching, first-aid for, 24

J

Jin Shin Do Foundation for Body-mind Acupressure, 86
Joint Fuel, 202
Journal writing, for stress relief, 223

Juice, apple vs. orange, 190
Juniper as diuretic, 131

K

Kava-kava, for anxiety, 207
Ketoprofen, 22
Kola nut, caffeine in, 131
Konjak, glucomannan in, 132

L

Lactation, body fat and, 116
Laparoscopic surgery, outpatient, 39
Laparoscopies, 38
Laparotomies, 39
Laughter, immune system and, 216–17
Lavender, in aromatherapy, 88
Laxatives, herbal, 131
LDL. *See* Cholesterol levels
Lipid profiles, 16
Lipton Soothing Moments Herbal Teas,
    222
Listening, active. *See* Active listening
Longevity
    childbearing and, 27
    exercise and, 138
    self-esteem and, 231
Love
    health benefits of, 218
    sustaining, 246–51
Low-density lipoproteins. *See* Cholesterol
    levels
Low-fat foods, 162
Lubriderm, 24
Lunch, energy levels and, 102
Lung cancer, selenium and, 200
Lupron (Rx), 39
Lupus, 14–15

M

Magnesium, 199–200
Makeup. *See* Cosmetics
Mammograms, 2, 3, 11–12, 44
    physical comfort during, 50
    reasons women don't have, 49–51

Mania, 106
Margarine, 188–89, 189
Marriage(s)
    maintaining healthy, 247–51
    male moodiness in, 252–56
    proposals, by women, 247
    sex in, 257–62
Massage
    foot, 222
    for headaches, 90
    scalp, 90, 264, 265, 279–80
Maté, caffeine in, 131
Mayonnaise, 121
Meat, grades of, 123
Medical foods, 194
Medications. *See also specific types*
    colors of, 20
    instructions for taking, 22
    over-the-counter, 19–25
Melatonin, 106, 203–4
Menopause. *See also* Estrogen
            replacement therapy (ERT);
            Hormone replacement therapy
            (HRT)
    early, 33
    fibroids and, 34
    heredity and, 44, 46
    smoking and, 46
    weight gain and, 116
Menstruation
    cramps during, 23
    heavy bleeding during
        alternative treatments for, 37–38, 41
        anemia from, 34, 102
        from fibroids, 34
        hysterectomies for, 2, 3, 36–37
    migraines during, 22
Mental health
    of mothers, 239
    walking and, 147
Meridia (Rx), 128–30
Metabolism, 114–15
    herbs to increase, 131
    low-calorie diets and, 102
Mexican yam, 208
Micronor (Rx), 41
Migraine headaches, 83–84. *See also*
            Headaches
    amnesia and, 258
    diet and, 86, 196–97
    green apple scent and, 83
    magnesium and, 200
    medications for, 22, 82, 84

PET scans, for mood lability, 254–55
Phototherapy, for allergies, 73
Phytochemicals, 184, <u>185</u>
PID, 14
Pill, the. *See* Contraceptives, oral
Plastic surgery. *See* Cosmetic surgery
Poison ivy, 25
Pokeroot, for endometriosis, 41
Polysporin, 24
Positron-emission tomography scans, for
    mood lability, 254–55
Posture
    headaches and, <u>91</u>
    for walking, 148
Potassium, in juices, 190
Precancers, cervical and uterine, <u>40</u>
Pregnancy
    ectopic, 14
    heredity and, <u>44</u>, <u>45–46</u>
    iron deficiency and, 103
Pregnenolone, 204
Prepackaged foods, 126, <u>194</u>
Progesterone
    for abnormal bleeding, 37, 41
    energy levels and, 104–5
Prostate, enlarged, 206
Prostate cancer, selenium and, 200
Protein deficiency, 182
Proteins, energy levels and, 102
Provera (Rx), 41
Prozac (Rx), 255
Psoriasis, 24
Psychological problems, of mothers, 239
Psyllium, 23
Pumpkin pie, <u>197</u>
Pushup, *156*

Q

Quad tightener, *154*
Quizzes
    beauty, <u>264–65</u>
    cosmetic surgery, <u>286–88</u>
    health know-how, <u>2–3</u>
    mother-daughter health links, <u>44–46</u>
    nutrition, <u>182–83</u>
    perfectionism, <u>232–33</u>
    personality, <u>108–11</u>
    relationships, <u>244–45</u>
    stress, <u>214–15</u>
    weight loss, <u>108–11</u>

R

Race
    heart disease and, 63
    osteoporosis and, 65
Raloxifene (Rx), <u>3</u>, 26–31, 72
Reaction time, low-calorie diet and, <u>166</u>
Reading, for stress relief, 223
Rebound headaches, <u>89</u>, 91
Red-laser phototherapy, for allergies,
    73
Red light, effect on exercise performance,
    122
Redux (Rx), 128
Relationships
    maintaining healthy, 247–51
    male moodiness in, 252–56
    quiz, <u>244–45</u>
Relaxation exercises, 172, 222
Renova (Rx), 276
Resistance training
    bone mass and, 68
    for weight loss, 137
Retin-A (Rx), 276
Riboflavin, 192
Robitussin Maximum Strength Cough,
    21
Rolfing, for headaches, 87
Rolf Institute, 87

S

St.-John's-wort, for depression, 207
Salad dressing, 119
Salicyclic acid creams, <u>287</u>
Saliva tests
    for breast cancer, <u>52</u>
    for stress, <u>224</u>
Salt, 124, 132
Sassafras, 208
Saw palmetto, for enlarged prostates,
    206
Scalpels, obsidian, <u>284</u>
Selective estrogen receptor modulators
    (SERMs), 26, 29
Selenium, cancer and, 200
Self-esteem
    longevity and, <u>231</u>
    mothers and, 238–39, 241–42
Senna as laxative, 131

T

W

Waist/hip ratio, heart disease and, 60, 62–63
Waist measurements, health risks and, 169
Walking
  benefits of, 145–47
  posture for, 148
  shoes for, 147–48
  tips for, 148–51, 151
Water, drinking
  benefits of, 209, 211–12
  energy levels and, 102
  during illness, 193
  weight loss and, 120, 123, 124, 168
Weight. *See also* Obesity
  gender and, 116–17
  heredity and, 44, 45, 114
  ideal, 169
  premenstrual, 113
Weight-bearing exercises, osteoporosis and, 67–68
Weight loss, 118–27
  chromium and, 202
  diet pills for, 128–30
  diets, unhealthy, 113–14
  eating habits and, 118–26, 167–68
  excuses and solutions, 159–64
  exercise and, 115, 134–37
  food smells and, 119
  herbs, 130–33, 133
  low-calorie diets and, 102, 166
  maintaining, 116, 137
  motivation for, 113, 160–61, 163
  personality and, 108–11
  plateaus, 114, 165–69, 167
  quiz, 108–11
  reaction time and, 166

sabotage by family members, 174–79, 176
Wrinkles
  eliminating, 274
  facial exercises and, 264
  preventing, 268, 275–76
  sleep and, 264, 265, 268, 271, 275, 287

X

Xenical (Rx), 130

Y

Yarrow, for heavy bleeding, 41
Yeast infections, 23–24
  home test for, 12
Yellowdock, for hormonal balance, 92
Yogurt
  bacteria in, 183, 195
  frozen, vs. ice cream, 191
  with fruit, 191
  for weight loss, 126
Yohimbe, 208

Z

Zanamivir (Rx), 80
Zantac 75, 23
Zinc
  calcium and, 65, 71
  for colds, 78
  sources of, 65, 190, 192